2nd Edition
Revised and Updated

NUTRITIONALLY
ncorrect

Why the Modern Diet
is Dangerous and
How to Defend Yourself

Allan N. Spreen, M.D., C.N.C.

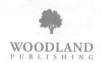

WOODLAND
PUBLISHING

The CIP record for this book is available from the Library of Congress.

For ordering information, contact:
Woodland Publishing, P.O. Box 160, Pleasant Grove, Utah 84062
(800) 777-2665

Note: The information in this book is for educational purposes only and is not recommended as a means of diagnosing or treating an illness. All matters concerning physical and mental health should be supervised by a health practitioner knowledgeable in
treating that particular condition. Neither the publisher nor author directly or indi-
rectly dispenses medical advice, nor do they prescribe any remedies or assume any
responsibility for those who choose to treat themselves.

ISBN 1-58054-325-1

10 9 8 7 6 5 4 3 2 1

Printed in the United States of America

Please visit our website:
www.woodlandpublishing.com

Dedication

To my parents, who put up with more than they should have had to; to my sister Cathy, without whom none of this would have happened; and especially to my sister Nancy, who I hope is watching from a comfortable perch up there somewhere.

Contents

Preface

THIS IS NOT a cookbook. But fear not. Though I'm not into reinventing the wheel, you'll learn where the best wheels can be found. We'll list a lot of them, cookbooks and otherwise.

The basic problem today in achieving good health does not lie in the measuring cup; it's more fundamental than that. If you don't even know which items in a given recipe are slowly killing you or sapping your quality of life, then each recipe becomes another game of Russian roulette with your health. (OK, it isn't quite that bad, maybe it's musical chairs?)

My practice constantly reinforced the presence of a recurring theme in nutrition and nutrition therapies. It ran along the lines of "how do I begin?" or "how can I get my husband (or my kids, or whoever) started in nutrition?"

Once you know what you're looking for, you can open any cookbook, scan a few pages, and know in seconds whether it's a health-promoting set of recipes. You can read any label, on any foodstuff, and know if you're being "had."

That's what this book is about, and that's my reason for writing it.

Trouble with
the Modern Diet

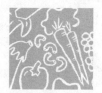

CHAPTER 1

Good Health: Mission Possible

IT DOESN'T TAKE a genius to get healthy. And it doesn't require you to be an all-out health nut. It just takes a little eye opening— a little pertinent information, if you will. Unfortunately, we as a population are being misled about the dangers to our health and just what we can do about it.

New Health Concerns

Look around you. For the first time in history, overweight people now outnumber the rest of the population of the United States—we'll use that country as representative of a "civilized" nation. (AP release, Oct. 16, 1996). One third of the population is twenty or more pounds overweight. Why? Aren't we more conscious about "low fat" than ever before? Aren't we watching our cholesterol levels closer than ever before? Aren't there far more people exercising than ever before? (Even if *we* aren't the ones exercising, everybody *else* should be skinny.) Not that many years ago, our relatives were noticeably slimmer than we are—without counting a single fat gram. There were no drugs to lower choles-terol or triglycerides, and the current "fitness movement" was nowhere to be seen. Now everyone panics if cholesterol breaks 200, and you can't find an empty machine at the fitness center.

This is not a sudden change over the last year or so (though the trend certainly seems to be continuing). In 1955, dietary fat intake in the United States was about 33 percent of total calories, while the number of overweight individuals was less than 25 percent of the total population. By 1990, the fat intake had decreased to under 25 percent, while the overweight population increased to 41 percent (Alfred 1995). So there's more to this situation than watch-ing fat grams (no matter what we're told on television), and it even looks like we're watching fat the wrong way!

There are more problems with our health than just weight gain: heart disease is increasing, and cancer is rampant. At a recent health seminar, a Canadian Ph.D. in cancer research stated that one in every three of us is getting cancer, and one in six will die of it! If he's even close to correct in his figures, there's a problem here. In an article called "Did You Know? . . ." by the publishers of *Prevention Magazine,* they explained: "Almost nobody got cancer or heart disease before 1905. The first heart attack was described in the *Journal of the American Medical Association* in 1908. In fact, if you look in a medical book from the 1860s, you won't find any-thing on coronary atherosclerosis (hardening of the arteries)."

Let's look at life expectancy statistics for the U.S. If you remove infant mortality rates, adults are now dying earlier than they used to, in the most technologically advanced medical system on the planet.

Some of the latest available data on life expectancy comes from the World Health Organization, which has ranked life expectancy using a new system called the Disability Adjusted Life Expectancy, or DALE. This is an attempt to take into account life span of healthy individuals separate from the effects of accidents and injuries (see sidebar on following page).

Check out all the arthritis victims hobbling around. Though they haven't yet died, many look awfully close to it. Stop for a sec-ond on the street, and consider some of the people using handicapped parking stickers. (Consider also lending a hand.) Even ignoring those who don't deserve the special status, it is becoming clearer that we are not aging gracefully as a population.

The Plan

What is going on here? Have we missed something, and, if so, can something be done about it? Probably a closer-to-home ques-

Disability Adjusted Life Expectancy Rankings

(Source: World Health Organization release, 4 June 2000)

RANK	AGE
1. Japan	74.5
2. Australia	73.2
3. France	73.1
4. Sweden	73.0
5. Spain	72.8
6. Italy	72.7
7. Greece	72.5
8. Switzerland	72.5
9. Monaco	72.4
10. Andorra	72.3
*	*
12. Canada	72.0
*	*
14. United Kingdom	71.7
*	*
*	*
*	*
*	*
22. Germany	70.4
*	*
24. United States	70.0

tion would be: Assuming that something can be done, just how much would you have to do to avoid this deteriorating quality and quantity of life? You already count fat grams, and maybe you've made a bunch of other sacrifices. Just what else do you have to do and how miserable do you have to get?

Obviously I believe something can be done—or this book wouldn't exist. (I believe it strongly.) It's happened "before my very eyes" too many times to ignore, with parents, kids, the elderly—you name it. It's also happened with my own body. However, if you are a beginner and at are least willing to consider a few changes, you stand to make great strides in improving your health.

In addition, I don't believe the changes required are really all that tough, and not just because I'm some kind of incredibly strong-willed health nut. I cheat with what I eat, and I enjoy myself; but I always remain aware of what goes in my mouth and its potential effects. That, and the fact that I feel worse when I cheat makes it easier to be "good." Being well informed makes all the difference. (I also use the term "health insurance," meaning a series of well-chosen supplements, but we're getting ahead of ourselves.)

There's another reason I'm confident these changes are well within the will power of most of us: Many people are applying will power to accomplish *unnecessary* tasks. Besides being well informed, there's another facet to making transitions to good health easier, and that is to make sure that your information is truly information and not *mis*information. You, of course, can't be absolutely guaranteed that my information is any less misinformation than the next guy's. However, my attempt at a guarantee is to stay as basic as possible in everything we discuss, so you can make your own decisions.

I'm not smart enough to reinvent the wheel, so I won't try. There are too many functional wheels out there; we don't need new ones. We need to understand why the old ones worked so well and why "wonder drug" cures are never going to happen. If you can drop the mindset of "soon they're going to have that disease cured," you'll be in a position to understand the powerful fundamentals of what's really going on and what you can do about it.

And I do mean that you can beneficially alter the health issues affecting your own body. Remember, no one cares as much about your body as you do. You have a responsibility here that you cannot afford to delegate.

My main concern about information versus misinformation is this: some of the things you might assume you need to do to get healthy you may not, in fact, need to do at all.

That can make things easier.

As an example, I pose a question: Have you found, or do you know, anyone—anyone—who feels that a low-fat diet is the easiest way to lose weight? Forget "easiest." Do you know anyone who feels it's even a useful way to lose weight? If there were any loss at all, I'll bet the dieter was doing something else at the same time.

The reason is simple, and no one can call it misinformation—like much of what is tossed out as gospel concerning low-fat diets. We're talking about an established biological fact available to any high school science class. No knowledgeable doctor or scientist will deny that sugars, starches, and proteins all convert, and readily so, to fat! You can eat a zero-fat diet, *zero percent* (now there's something hard to do), but unless you eat less than you use for energy and repair, you will gain weight and that weight will be fat. Every second-semester freshman medical student knows that, or he or she won't pass physiology class.

Not only that, low fat doesn't taste good. So, nearly all the new, highly advertised low-fat foods are made to taste good by loading them with, guess what, sugar.

Why aren't we told stuff like that in all this low-fat hoopla? None of it is arguable. It's out there, on the labels, and in the textbooks; not subject to any sort of debate. (I'm sure someone will find a way, but let's generalize.) Is it possible we're getting a little misinformation?

Anyway, that's the sort of thing I'm getting at. It's possible that the water you drink could have more to do with lowering your cholesterol than your low-fat diet. How tough a change would that be, compared to counting all those fat grams?

Start with the Basics

To start with the basics, the approach here will introduce you to the concept of "nutrient density." Hopefully it won't be so in depth to bore you, but certainly enough to reinforce its vital nature. In this day and age, nutrient-dense foods are difficult to get, while their importance can not be understated. Once you learn to focus your diet on such foods, the game becomes much simpler.

Okay, so that's how we're going to approach health. This book is designed for the beginner, so if you're a hotshot health-nut type, you may find this information somewhat elementary. However, the last section does contain recommendations for the next steps, in whatever direction you wish to take (unless I run you off completely).

That's the approach. Again, though, why bother? What's in it for you? Statistics are just numbers, so let's get closer to home: Do you feel okay? Are there things you want to accomplish that you're too tired to handle? Is there a family history of health problems? Do you look in the mirror and cringe at what you see? Do you write off your undesirable symptoms as just "the aging process"? Do you have some chronic illness?

Whatever the reason, what you don't know can make you sick—for real. What you're up against is a media blitz that has become aware that you aren't worth much money when you're well. It's the opposite for farm animals and pets. They aren't worth much when they're sick. There's real money in sick people, though, whether losing something in an operation, swallowing something for "acid indigestion" or that "pounding headache," or just painting something on the ol' hemorrhoid. This book will introduce you to the health information necessary to start undoing the damage that years of health misinformation can cause. You can avoid the stresses you have been heaping upon your body, if you just know about them.

Not only that, you'd be surprised how much simpler it is than you might think to feel better. Once the education is there, it's like seeing foods (and their labels) for the first time. Your decisions become much easier. Even how you eat (which is free), once it becomes a habit, can have you feeling better within days. If that happens, the changes promote themselves. You'll not only keep the changes, you'll forget that they've now become an integral part of your life. Even my eight-year-old niece voluntarily avoided ice cream, once she learned it was responsible for making her feel ill. I could hardly believe it myself.

Step-by-Step Information

So, we're going to start at the beginning. If you're impatient, and you just want the program, you can turn to Chapter 20 and get started. I hope, if you're a beginner, that you don't do it that way. It's quicker, sure, but like any "quick fix" it's missing the foundation that tends to help make it permanent. If you really understand why you are changing something, the hassle of change is reduced, and much more likely to be incorporated into the way you think about your health from now on.

The chapters are ordered in such a way that you are first introduced to the problems in our diet that can adversely affect our health. This is not meant to scare you (too much). It's to show you just how close to home the problem areas can be, and what basic things can be done about them.

Then we'll take a look at an important technique for handling these stresses, offering some protection from those we can't possibly avoid. Can a nutritional supplement plan really provide a nutritional "insurance policy" that can do such a thing? If you become convinced that it can, then you'll want to know how best to evaluate your own policy. Once you understand the "fine print" (sometimes literally), you can better protect both your health and your pocketbook.

Once we cover what we're up against and how to start defending ourselves in general, then we can put the whole package together for an integrated approach that can become a way of life, instead of a daily hassle.

Through examples and repetition the philosophy will hopefully start to ingrain itself, or at least parts of it will. This is not a "program" as such. There's no selling our own lines of vitamins, foods, athletic gear, or anything. This is information only, supplied to help you enjoy life on this planet by feeling as good as possible. I hate to think of the guidelines as "rules," which is what they will look like if you don't understand the rationale. That's why I hope you'll read from start to finish.

See what you think, and give it a try for just one month. No tricks, no gimmicks, no product sales pitch. Plain, tested, useful data that can help you feel better, and then, after you feel the difference these changes make in your health, you can move on to whatever next steps you feel inclined to try.

CHAPTER 2

Sugar: Sweet Poison

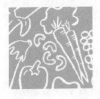

A BIT MELODRAMATIC? Maybe. After all, we're not talking arsenic or fluoride, or something that will drop you in your tracks. The subject here is merely sugar—plain, everyday, pure, white sugar. I eat it. In fact, I grew up addicted to it. I still cringe to think about it.

However, sugar really is a killer. No, it won't kill you this instant, but you should respect what's happening because, slowly maybe, it'll get you. Really. Compared to our ancestors, we are eating vast amounts of sugar. Some experts say it's over 125 pounds per person per year in the U.S. (I'll bet it's higher.)

These days, everyone seems to think in calories; that is, a calorie is a calorie is a calorie. Eat too many, you gain weight, not too many, you don't. I've heard some of my colleagues, and even some of my old medical school professors, say the same thing. There's a well-known health/exercise speaker on national public radio in the U.S. who has some excellent information, but he says the same thing. I don't buy it—not exactly. This is a bit more than just a question of semantics. Allow me to defend myself.

A Calorie Is a Calorie Is a Calorie . . .

Okay, if you want to get technical (ugh), a calorie is a unit of energy—heat energy. It is the amount of energy required to increase the temperature of a certain amount of water, a certain degree, under certain conditions. (In the human body, we usually deal with 1,000-calorie amounts, which are Calories with a capital "C.") In the laboratory, such controlled experiments are carried out using calorimeters, devices designed to measure such things.

Using this argument, obviously a calorie, as a definition, does not change. It's a unit of energy, and that's it. The problem is, in the real world, we are not a bunch of calorimeters, existing at standard temperature and pressure in an experimental laboratory. As human organisms there are differences, and some are big ones. These differences from the experimental model have to do both with how calories are packaged and how the body deals with those packages.

The major types of packaging are proteins, fats, and carbohydrates, but right this moment these are not our focus. Rather, let's deal with a subset of the carbohydrate package, that of the simple carbohydrate, as opposed to the complex. In fact, our real issue here is even a subset of that, taking us down to the refined simple carbohydrate, as opposed to the unrefined. (A similar issue exists in the complex carbohydrate subset. See Chapter 3.)

The simple carbohydrates are the sugars. These are mostly sweet-tasting substances of similar chemistries, such as glucose (dextrose), sucrose, fructose, lactose, galactose, etc., with each containing the same number of calories per unit of weight. (I know, a calorie is a calorie is a . . .)

In nature, these sugars are found, with one notable exception, in an unrefined state, such as in sugar cane, sugar beets, and most fruits, where they are pretty sweet naturally. In other sources, such as corn, rice, and even milk, where unless something is done to them, they are not so sweet. Almost all vegetables and fruits have fair amounts of natural sugar in them; and whether naturally sweet or not so sweet, there is little problem eating basically as much of them as desired (not counting food allergies, but we'll get to that later).

Then man gets into the act.

The "Naked" Calorie

This is where things start to happen. If you have ever gone out into a field of sugar cane, cut out a piece of the moist core, and sampled it, you know that it is appreciably sweet, but it's nothing compared with the taste of "pure-cane sugar" in the form of those beautiful crystals you would buy at the store.

I believe that there would be little or no problem eating either sugar cane or sugar beets, as a squeezed, nonconcentrated juice straight from the plant, even over the long haul. (I'm sure you could get carried away, somehow, or you could be allergic, but aside from that.) First of all, every nutrient required for the assimilation (absorption and utilization) of the juice is contained within it. If you chew the stalk, you even get natural fiber. This seems to be a law of nature. A real food contains within itself the nutrients required for its use by the body. The exceptions to this rule have to do with biochemical individuality, meaning how each person's body is genetically predisposed to handle different foods.

The point here is that sugar, real sugar, is not the problem. The problem is that refined sugar no longer qualifies as food. This means that when "the white stuff" is ingested, the vitamins, and particularly the minerals required for burning (or storing) that fuel internally (B1, B2, biotin, niacin, pantothenic acid, magnesium, and others), do not accompany the now totally pure and concentrated sugar! The body will handle the fuel, but it does it by taking from body stores already in existence. These stores, of course, were supplied from whole foods previously eaten. What happens if too much "food" is eaten of the "take" variety, and not enough of the "give" variety? You can see where this is headed.

Long-term diets of "naked" calories like those in refined sugar continually stress the body by sapping it of its internal stores of nutrients. Eventually, deficiencies arise, possibly of a subclinical nature, or possibly of a combined nature, such that they do not fit the textbook descriptions of deficiency states. I believe this is happening on a daily basis in this country. Most of our diets are full of naked, nonfood substances. It's a slow—but harmful—even deadly process.

The Concentrated Calorie

Sorry, sugar lovers, there's more. This standard calorie is not only naked, but it's also concentrated. Besides the nutrients being removed, the water is all gone; the juice is now a crystal. Soluble fiber is also missing. (This is even more pronounced in fruit when it's converted to fruit juice, then even worse as it's refined to pure fructose, or fruit sugar. It's also an issue in high-fructose corn syrup.)

William Dufty, in his book, *Sugar Blues*, reveals just how concentrated our processed sugar really is. He found that the equivalent of five ounces of refined sugar requires two and a half pounds of sugar beets! That much sugar is nothing for most people to eat in a day (even in ten minutes!). Try it with the beets. Nature builds in its own controls, which we have perverted, for whatever reason. Instead, we are left with a concentrate that has little to do with the original sugar cane or beets.

This concentrated substance is 100 percent pure sugar, and no matter what they say on television, it is in no way "natural." It's a chemical—basically a drug. Pure dextrose is even classified as a drug in hospitals, both as an intravenous and oral treatment for insulin excess.

We can get this marvelous stuff, however, over the counter. Apparently, killing yourself is legal, as long as the poison is slow enough. Part of this slow process involves the body's mechanism for handling the simple carbohydrate package. Once sugar enters the system, the blood sugar rises. The body's response to this is to squirt a little insulin into the bloodstream to remove the sugar from the blood, and send it to the muscle and brain cells (or somewhere else, if you don't happen to be lifting or thinking enough).

Here's an aside for you weight-conscious people who count fat grams. Sugar that is not used in the body is not passed out (unless you have diabetes and pee out calories as sugar—a rather poor way to lose weight). It's stored, and it's not stored as sugar. It is converted and stored as fat! So, you can cut your fat grams to zero, but if you eat too much concentrated carbohydrate instead, you put on fat. The low-fat advertisers didn't tell you that? Hmmm. Remember this; we'll be coming back to it.

Now, back to our show. If the sugar the body receives is unnaturally concentrated, the pancreas (the insulin-secreting organ) can overreact and secrete too much insulin too fast. Instead of a slow decrease of blood sugar, this causes your blood sugar to drop too quickly. When this happens, the level usually goes too low, too quickly. The body tries to compensate by breaking out stored sugar in the form of glycogen to get the level back up, but before that happens, something else occurs: You feel bad. This is called reactive hypoglycemia. The blood sugar drops fast enough to cause a myriad of symptoms, including headaches, irritability, fatigue, abdominal pains, and even muddled thinking, blurred vision, and depression.

It causes one other thing: cravings. Your body quickly learns that the key to feeling better fast is a concentrated sugar "fix." It may be a doughnut, candy bar, cup of coffee (either loaded with sugar or with a substitute fix of caffeine); whatever, but it usually will be a simple carbohydrate, if not a refined one, because the sugar release is faster. The quicker the release, the faster the blood sugar goes back up and the faster you feel better.

The problem with this process is you went back up too fast, so you have caused the same problem all over again, setting yourself up for another fall an hour or so later. This "roller-coaster" effect is a vicious cycle that traps carbohydrate addicts. I believe it is depressingly common. (Years ago, "reactive hypoglycemia" was held to be strictly a quack term and called the "nondisease." Now, it is fairly common to hear it even from conventional physicians.)

Reactive hypoglycemia is not really a disease. It's a symptom. It just leads to disease.

The Killer Package

The concentrated, naked calorie, that's the killer package, and we have discussed the body's standard response to it. Biochemical individuality dictates that different people will react differently to this stress, but all the reactions will be unpleasant to some degree—you may be just a little tired until the sugar comes back up; on the other hand you may experience a major behavioral change, or something else. Avoid the package. It's a time bomb. And it's everywhere.

Once you decide to make the effort to stay away from refined sugar, actually pulling it off may be even tougher than you think, due to the fact that it's in almost everything we eat. For example, it would seem to be a logical decision to buy raw sugar, so that you could get all the nutrients from the sugar cane even though the water has been removed. The problem is, you are a few decades too late. Years ago, raw sugar truly was raw sugar. Now it's just white sugar with a tan. "Brown" sugar, for example, used to be heavy, dark, rich, moist, distinctly flavored, and difficult to get out of the box. (It took a chisel if it sat out too long.) Now, however, apparently for our convenience and protection (real brown sugar was said to be contaminated), the actual definition of "brown sugar" has been changed. "Brown" sugar now means granulated, refined sugar that has been colored by adding back in some molasses. Even if you try to play the game better, someone changes the rules on you!

Probably the closest thing to natural sugar you can get nowadays is turbinado sugar, available in health food stores. This is basically a compromise substance, still granulated and refined, but the refining is not quite complete. In other countries worldwide natural sugars may be available, but know what you are looking for.

True blackstrap molasses is where the nutrients in refined sugar went, including appreciable amounts of natural iron, calcium, magnesium, and the B-vitamins. Once all of the sweet part is totally removed, what is left is the blackstrap. You could, in fact, reconstitute refined sugar by mixing the two together, but what a hassle.

Light molasses is not the same thing. Some of the sugar part remains, and some of the nutrient parts have been removed. The darker the better, if you decided to go this route.

To really avoid the stress and degenerative disease I believe are caused by sugar, abstinence is probably the only way. (Don't worry! I mean abstinence from sugar!)

The Killer Response

The magnitude of the rise of "adult-onset" (also called type II) diabetes in the last half century is mind blowing. This is no longer a rare disease, as it once was. Is there a connection between this disease and concentrated sugar? I believe that there is.

Depending on the body's constitution, at some point the pancreas, which has been tormented by the endless stress of these refined sugar "whippings," can decide to call a halt. It gets the signal to respond to high sugar, but it's just too tired, so it lets the high blood sugar stay there, and you are diabetic. Maybe you can control it with diet, maybe you can't. It depends on the stress and how you respond to it.

You absolutely must avoid the package that started the mess. Some people need drugs, some even need injections. Often, supplementation helps lower the amount of medication you might need; you might be able to come off it altogether, if things haven't gotten too bad. Besides a diet high in protein, with only complex carbohydrates, instead of the simple ones, the addition of chromium, vanadium, B-complex and vitamin C can be very helpful.

Nature's Refined Carbohydrate

We can't leave the subject of refined sugar without mentioning nature's little refinery, the honeybee. These little guys (oops, gals) actually refine sugar because they concentrate it really well. Some types of honey are better than others. Tupelo honey contains the most fructose over sucrose (table sugar). Since this sweetener takes longer to be used in the system, this is considered a plus, as the pancreas has a little longer to respond. Also, fructose tastes sweeter than sucrose, so you don't need as much. Bear in mind that this is still a sugar, so honey is not a license to steal. Taken straight it's sticky, which can make trouble in the tooth decay department, plus sugar-sensitive people may have to avoid it anyway.

The difference is that honey—real, raw honey—has calories that are not naked. Raw honey is packed with enzymes, minerals, vitamins, and other things unique to honey, many of which have been revered for centuries, much longer than most of our miracle drugs. Get the darkest you can find, and include the comb if possible.

Please note I said *raw* honey. There is a trick here. Honey that does not say "raw" is heated, and the heat destroys all sorts of good stuff. Even "uncooked" honey is heated, just not as high. (If you don't heat honey, it crystallizes in big, expensive packaging machines, and of course we can't have that.)

There is another reason to seek dark, raw honey. The major manufacturers want consistently light color and minimal flower taste for uniformity. It is not hard to do. The trick is to take refined, white sugar, dissolve it in water, and leave it at the door of the hive, so the bees aren't tempted to go elsewhere. (Sly, dirty trick, as far as I'm concerned.) Most honey you see on grocery store shelves is made this way, and it obviously cannot have all of the nutritional aspects of honey gathered from flowers, so beware when you shop.

Two excellent information sources on honey are *Honey And Your Health,* by B.F. Beck, M.D., and *Honey I Love You,* by Rev. Maurice Ness. If you are going to eat sugar, do it this way. (Rev. Ness even has recipes.)

What are the Alternatives?

The best switch, assuming you can't quit sweets, is to convert to simple, unrefined carbohydrates. These are the fruits, any fruit. Try to eat the whole fruit and avoid dried fruits, as you can eat a higher volume without the liquid in there. Beware of fruit juice, too, since you can drink more fruit than you can eat.

Okay, so you just cannot give up the sweet taste completely, and you need something to add to foods. Is there anything you can do about avoiding the naked calorie while still enjoying a sweet taste?

Actually there are a few possibilities, but each has its drawbacks. One option is a sweetener called stevia, a little-known herbal agent that some health food stores carry. It's hard to find, and long-term effects are not really known, but I bet they are far better than refined sugar. This stuff is really sweet, much more than sugar is, so you don't need much, but it's not cheap. Personally, I like this choice best.

Another option is xylitol, a relatively new sweetener that does not require insulin to be used by the body. Its long-term effects are not yet well studied, but some research suggests it is okay for teeth.

Among artificial products probably the most noteworthy item is aspartame (the most popular brand name is Nutrasweet). It's sweet and readily available, but you have to be careful. There are reports that the product can break down in the human body to toxic chemicals that can cause not only symptoms but also actual damage, including neurological illnesses that can be difficult to undo. The outcry is so extensive that there are many sources of information publicizing the advantages of avoiding this stuff, and the topic has grown too big to adequately cover in a beginner's guide. However, if you use this chemical at all, I'd suggest a review of the work done at the Aspartame Consumer Safety Network, (http://web2.airmail.net/marystod), P.O.Box 78064, Dallas, Texas, 75738, (phone 241-352-4368). There's also an independent web site report on it at www.holisticmed.com/aspartame/. It's not something I'd use.

Also in the artificial arena, saccharin seems to have less side effects than aspartame and contains no calories. It is a synthetic chemical, however, so who knows what's going on in the body over years of use? Sucaryl™, which is a cyclamate, is not legal in this country due to cyclamate research funded by an organization with a high potential for ulterior (i.e., pro-sugar) motives. This is the best tasting of the artificials and requires the least amount for sweetening, but if you are not in Mexico or Canada, you cannot get it. Again, it is synthetic.

The best sweetener, healthwise, is FOS, which stands for "fructo-oligo-saccharides" (wow). This is extremely beneficial for the intestinal tract, as it stimulates the growth of good bacteria. The downsides, unfortunately, are that it's expensive, only half as sweet as sugar, and breaks down at high temperatures. (It also can cause temporary gas in a person with yeast in the G.I. tract.)

There is now a new sweetener called Sucralose (i.e., brand name Splenda). It's sweeter than sugar, has no calories, and isn't broken down by heat. It's actually made from sugar, but chlorine atoms are substituted for other atoms in the original molecule. I don't trust the use of chlorine for much of anything regarding human consumption. The manufacturer maintains that this is a completely unabsorbed molecule, but there seems to be some controversy over whether that's really true. For more information to help you make up your own mind, consider the web site www.holisticmed.com/splenda/. In my opinion, the final word on this unique sweetener isn't in yet.

Good information worth studying concerning all sorts of sweeteners may be found at www.holisticmed.com/sweet/.

Maybe you can't win, but it's sure worth it to keep on trying.

A Final Word

As a sugar addict, trying hard to stay "on the wagon," I know for many people avoiding the stuff is very difficult. It is worth the effort, however. A few days off sugar, especially for someone who eats tons of it, can make you feel much better. Also, the harder it is to quit, the better you will probably feel if you can pull it off. Those who end up feeling the best are those who quit for two to four days, and at that point feel worse. Hang on, if that happens. Most likely you are in withdrawal, and you are almost guaranteed some degree of improvement. You would hate to miss a health factor so simple and close to home if it really could help you start to feel better.

If you are one of the "sugar people," I truly hope you will give these thoughts a try. If you've gotten this far, you must have enough interest in health improvement to give it a shot. It's one step in the right direction, and I don't think it's a small one.

CHAPTER 3

Our Daily Bread:
Staff of Life or Broken Crutch?

WHETHER RELIGIOUS OR NOT, just about everyone knows the term "staff of life" as a synonym for bread. The term is certainly appropriate. In the same way that a stout, hardwood staff would assist a traveler along a perilous, hard-trodden route, so this life-giving foodstuff has supported man for many thousands of years. It should still be the case.

Should be. Today, however, our staff of life is not providing the support it once did, not for the vast majority of consumers. For them, it barely qualifies as an old, broken crutch. The signs of that change are clearly showing in our health, for anyone who really cares to look; and it's time, way past time, for people to recognize that fact, because our health really is at stake.

The Issue

What is the problem here? The U.S. purports to be the most technologically advanced nation in the world. The output of the food processing industry is truly unsurpassed, with surplus food even sent to much of the rest of the world. The ability to generate huge quantities of food, extraordinary amounts, is unquestioned.

The question, as you most likely have guessed, is that of food quality. I am going to be so brazen as to suggest that the quality of one of our foods, bread, (worldwide) is generally so poor as to actually make the issue suitable for debate as to whether we can truly even classify our bread as food at all!

So we remain on the same wavelength, let's define our term:

Food: Anything which, when taken into the body, serves to nourish or build up the tissues or to supply body heat.
(*Dorland's Medical Dictionary,* 25th Ed.)

Food: That which is eaten or drunk or absorbed for the growth and repair of organisms and the maintenance of life.
(*New Illustrated Webster's Dictionary,* 1992)

I feel our standard bread only does one part of the above, specifically the supplying of body heat. The calories in bread do that, but with the "tissue build-up" part or the "organism repair" part, I just cannot agree. In fact, over the long haul (the short haul in guinea pig/rat experiments), I feel the opposite is happening. Tissues are breaking down and the organism is moving into a state of disrepair, such that life is not being maintained.

The Argument

Refined, white bread is suitable only for elementary school paste and paper maché. How can anyone say such a thing? The key is that today's bread is not the stuff our ancestors were eating 2,000 years ago, or even 200 years ago.

Bread is a carbohydrate, specifically a complex carbohydrate, as opposed to a simple one. As you know the simple carbohydrate category includes sugar, fruits—the sweet stuff. The complex category is the starches, which include grains, breads, cereals, pastas, potatoes, and other vegetables.

Unfortunately, both the simple and complex groups themselves have two subsets: the unrefined and the refined, and herein lies the crux of the problem. (For those who skip around in their reading, sugar and simple carbohydrates are described in Chapter 2.)

When unrefined, the grain is left totally in its original state, other than being dehulled (the inedible shell removed) and crushed. In this state, flour contains within itself all the nutrients required for its assimilation by the body, certainly a miracle of nature if there ever were one. In fact, there are usually excesses available so the body can add to its stores. This is borne out in controlled animal studies that show shortened lifespan and increased incidence of degenerative diseases when kept on a refined diet, while similar populations prosper and even reverse diseased conditions on an unrefined one. You want double-blind studies? They can't be done in a case like this, since it's too easy to tell the two diets apart, but at least the test animals are not subject to a placebo effect! (There are many similar situations.)

These removed nutrients are not limited to just vitamins, such as portions of the B-complex and vitamin E, but also minerals, such as iron, calcium, magnesium, manganese, zinc, and others, plus a large amount of the unsaturated fatty acids (which fat-gram-counting dieters need badly). There are more calories, more carbohydrates, and less protein in white flour compared to whole wheat. On top of that, before the refining process occurs, the flour is full of fiber, over seven times as much as the refined stuff, which is what makes unrefined bread heavy (really heavy, in everything but calories). Using other grains, the differences may be even greater.

I won't insult you by discussing whether having more natural vitamins and minerals is better than less, but what about all that fiber? Most of that is not even absorbed, so what difference could it make in a simple slice of bread? Tons.

If you are concerned about weight gain, I might even mean that literally. Fiber is a serious part of this argument. Remember that bread is a starch. This type of carbohydrate is composed of long chains of sugar molecules linked together by chemical bonds. The body breaks down these chains by destroying the linking bonds between the sugar molecules, using digestive enzymes, then it handles the sugar like any other sugar. The breakdown process starts even at the chewing process, with enzymes in the saliva, and continues through much of the upper digestive tract.

Fiber's first effect is to slow the mixing of enzymes with the starch, since the fiber is in the way. This slows the breakdown of starch to sugar. Therefore, sugar is more slowly released into the system. This allows a slow increase of blood sugar, rather than a fast increase. (Hang with me, now, I'm on a roll.) A situation of rising sugar in the blood tells the pancreas that it needs to crank up its production of insulin to bring down the blood sugar level, which is one of its jobs. (This is an effort to get the sugar out of the blood and into the muscle and brain cells.) The problem is that the sugar went up too fast, so the pancreas puts out too much insulin. When this happens, the blood sugar comes down too fast, and overshoots its normal low point, or at least gets there too quickly. At this point, symptoms are generated. This is reactive hypoglycemia, or low blood sugar as a delayed response to too much oral sugar, and you feel bad. Symptoms can be fatigue, irritability, temper flares, depression, abdominal pain, headaches, and others.

There's more. If the brain and muscles cannot utilize all this sugar at once, then the body does a really neat thing: it stores it. Guess how the body stores sugar it considers an excess. Other than a tiny bit stored as glycogen, the body stores excess sugar as fat. So, everyone you know who faithfully counts their fat grams has a problem: It is easily possible to eat zero grams of fat and put on large amounts of weight. That's how conscientious dieters get fat. The low-fat advertisers never told them they were making their own by eating most of the low-fat foods, which are laced with sugar for taste purposes. Cute, huh?

Believe it or not, there's even more. This huge amount of fiber that has been removed does something else: It fills you up, without adding a calorie. Bread made with real, unrefined flour is incredibly filling. Then, on top of that, it makes you thirsty and absorbs water like a sponge. You just can't eat as much of this type of bread, even if you like it, so you have cut your caloric intake down even farther. (Not only that, it keeps you regular, and laxatives are at the very top of the demand chart for over-the-counter medications.)

What about the special case of the athlete, energy driven and looking for lots of carbohydrates? The situation is the same, even for those who need, or think they need, lots of "carbs." If the quick-energy calories these guys are ingesting are refined, they run into the same rapid high–rapid low sugar scenario. Unrefined, complex carbohydrates still offer rapid-release energy, so fats and proteins do not have to be broken down as early, while the "sugar slump" is avoided. Staying within the normal limits of the blood sugar cycle gives better sustained energy release. (Most high-stamina athletes have felt the sugar-slump, often without even knowing what it is. This is a big part of "the wall" that can cost them success.)

Distance athletes should, in fact, carbohydrate "load." (If you don't know the term, then you probably don't need it.) The loading, however, should be accomplished with unrefined whole grains, cereals, pastas, and breads, not sugar or white flour junk that breaks down too quickly.

Actually, there is more, but enough of the arguments. (We could discuss fecal matter and the mechanics of its progress through the intestinal tract, but not before dinner.) Why has this situation occurred? Why haven't those responsible for our food, or, if no one's responsible, those who profit by our purchase of food, done something about this foodstuff time bomb?

The Cause

If the previous section is even partially true (I have no reason to lie), why are we eating refined flour? It isn't really because it tastes better; we have just been programmed, for the most part, to think so. (I used to adore the stuff.) Part of it may be that it looks better, however. It is a beautiful, pure white. Unrefined, whole-grain flour almost looks dirty, with dark specks and heavy ground up particles in it. Plus, at the advent of the refining process, only the rich could afford white flour, so it became quite an ego trip to have it, causing whatever its taste was to catch on. But that still does not explain the origination of the process. Why would one bother in the very beginning? Originally, the equipment would be a huge capital outlay. Why?

Flour is refined for shelf life. Not *your* life. Shelf life. Most bugs won't eat the stuff (which may or may not say something about us.) It can be transported much further, even without refrigeration. Add a few preservatives (I don't really understand why they bother), and the stuff will look good for ages. It may squeeze fresh and look great, but don't think for a second your lab rats will do well on it—and so you might consider that you won't, either.

Are you aware that many cereal companies double as livestock feed companies? Chicken feed is whole grain, as are other feeds. Chickens can tell what is edible, for the most part, and what should be left. We get what's left. Chickens are not worth much when they are sick. (I guess we aren't worth much when we are well!) Once the real food is removed by the refining process, it is not thrown away. It can be valuable, and so it is marketed. Price a jar of wheat germ at the store sometime. That's what's supposed to be in your cereal and bread! Why do you have to pay (a lot) more for it?

There is probably one more reason: white flour certainly cooks better. Even most supposedly "whole-wheat" breads have white flour in them so they will rise better. I'm not a cook, but I have to admit that junk food pastries just aren't the same with the heavy stuff. Too bad.

Special Warnings

There are things you have to watch for, if you decide to care about any of this. One is that "whole-grain" flour may well be no such thing. To get true whole-wheat flour in the U.S., for example, the label has to read "100 percent stone ground whole wheat," and even then I've seen tricks pulled. Be careful. The heavy stuff is more expensive because it spoils, and it's harder to work with. Producers often try to slip a mixture over on you. Remember, all flour in regular white bread is wheat flour, so asking for wheat bread does not work. Some "whole-wheat" breads will use mostly white flour, add a small amount of unrefined flour, plus some molasses or something to darken it, and try to sell it to you for a higher price.

Bleached flour, used in the finest, lightest breads and pastries is the worst, because it is the most highly refined. How about rye bread? I'm guilty of this one. I love the taste, but this is refined, white flour with some rye seeds in it.

Pumpernickel is a tougher one. This was supposed to be 100 percent rye-flour bread, but somehow, when we weren't looking, they slipped the refined stuff in there, too. It may be heavy, and it may be dark, but it is not totally unrefined. Check the label. It's there.

Finally, we reach the ultimate fraud: "enriched" bread/flour. This word, to the enlightened, means nothing but refined, white flour, by definition. Nearly every flour in this country is enriched. There may be some ultra-fine pastry flours or something that are not enriched, but they are rare. In the "enrichment" process a tiny amount of a few synthetic vitamins, and nothing else, is added back into the flour after refining all the good stuff out. Forget the fiber, the minerals, other vitamins, and any micronutrients we might not even know about; they are not there. So, if you see "100 percent unbleached, enriched, wheat flour," don't kid yourself—it's refined white flour, nothing more.

Bear in mind that all of the above warnings apply equally to everything involved with grains, whether it be flour, bread, cereal, grain side dishes, or pastas of any type. Read labels, and you will find that a normal grocery store has almost no real, whole grains.

The Solution

If you decide to try this health-improvement method, your sources, as you've guessed, are limited. Your safest bet is a conscientious health food store that carries only real, unrefined, whole-grain foods. There are now more and more small bread shops that make their own bread. Most of them have a honey whole wheat that may fill the bill of really natural, but usually there is only one. You still have to read labels carefully, if you don't want to get stung, but you can consider this simple (fun) screening test: if you drop the loaf on your toe and it hurts, you're on the right track.

Concerning packaged grains, for side dishes, soups, etc., use brown rice instead of white; seek dehulled barley instead of pearled; try lesser-known grains that do not tend to be refined, like millet or amaranth. Look out for grits and hominy; they do not supply whole-grain support. Even "quick" oatmeal has had some processing help. Get whole oats, and do it the long way.

There is a huge variety of pastas in the health food stores: lasagna, spaghetti, angel hair, noodles, macaroni, the works. They are darker, heavier, require less to fill you up (remember that before you cook up a ton), and they are more expensive. You have to read carefully here, too. Some are only half whole grain, using mixed grains, or partially refined flours, and others are great. The available types include: whole wheat, artichoke, spinach, and brown rice. The tastes are different, but some are tolerable, even to kids. Angel-hair type is usually preferred as a spaghetti, since the pasta is heavier to start with, although the noodles are a bit thinner.

Parting Comments

Whether for yourself or your family, these types of changes can be a bit trying at times because they really are changes, and everyone fears losing the status quo. Unenlightened individuals are quick to rebel against spaghetti that's the green stuff, or bread that's heavy as a brick. Attempt to persevere, and try to educate those around you. At the same time, go to health food stores and continue to read about what is *real health*, and the advantages of true "health foods" and supplements. Don't let someone else tell you what you need or don't need, or even what is or is not quackery (including me). Check it out and then decide. The alternative is to play games with Mother Nature, and everyone knows what happens when you tick her off.

Read, try new foods, and be patient; it can take awhile to back off from the preferences for junk food, but the potential rewards may amaze you and make you wish you had done it years ago. Try it. I believe it's well worth the effort.

CHAPTER 4

Don't Drink the Water

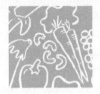

YOU TURN ON the faucet. From it issues forth crystal clear, cool, refreshing water. It's been processed by the local utilities, whose job it is to assure that we're provided with the best water possible. It's been purified, tested, treated, maintained, monitored and distributed right to our homes. It's reasonably priced and thoroughly convenient . . . Don't drink it.

So, you've put a water softener onto your incoming water line. Those hard water stains and crusts are gone. The rotten egg smell is gone. Your coffee tastes better. . . . Don't drink it.

One of my concerns has to include just how that water is purified. It is fundamental to understand, however, just how serious the the need is for strong water treatment. The main problem is not the one we hear so much about; i.e., the seepage into the ground of weird new chemicals. That makes for excellent press and allows for tons of grant money to be allocated for high-tech chemical research. That dilemma exists, no question, but the real, high-volume problem is not nearly as spectacular. It's a much more mundane, more expensive, more fundamental horror: Our own sewage is dumped directly into our rivers from every city in the nation. (The use of septic tanks is not the technique of cities!)

Think about it. Unless you are the absolute uppermost town on a river, your water intake is starting with all the dumped wastes of the town above you. And all the towns above them. Pleasant thought. We take someone else's sewage, draw it into our water supply, chop it up, filter it, dump enough chlorine into it to hopefully kill all the worms, microbes, and other bugs and parasites that are obviously there, and then we, uh . . . drink it.

A not uncommon misconception is that as long as all the "bugs" are gone everything is okay. Pump that chlorine or bromine in there, kill off all the bad guys, and everything is taken care of. Nothing could be so disastrously further from the truth.

It's true that microorganisms cause the most acute adverse effects, usually diarrhea. It would be nice, therefore, to be able to drink water without playing host to every *Giardia lamblia* or amoeba that comes out of the pipe. It's also true that we are being bombarded by huge quantities of chemicals, estimated at over 70,000 types, with hundreds more new pesticides, fertilizers, hormones, additives, industrial chemicals, and organic compounds coming at us each year, many of which leach into our water supply. Every water filter company is competing to convince you that it is the best at removing lead, benzene, or one of those chemicals no one can pronounce, like trichloromethylene or trihalomethane. At present, the problem is more fundamental.

The effort here is not to sell you a water filter, though I think you need one; my intention is to convince you that you should be very concerned about what is happening to our water and how serious a problem it really is. My next effort is to introduce you to a process and convince you of the need for that process. Once convinced, maybe together we can begin to push for a change in the way our water is treated before it is pumped to us.

In the end, we need a way to process out the bad bugs and nasty pollutants in the water without being killed by the process itself. This is the biggest danger we face by far because something has to be done to fix the water, besides spending fortunes on home filters and bottled water. It's sort of a "catch-22" at the moment: You need to process, but the processing kills you.

Danger #1

During the Vietnam War, autopsies on American soldiers killed in action showed incredibly high buildups of arteriosclerotic plaques throughout their vascular systems, as if they were far older than they appeared. Keep in mind that these soldiers were the country's finest physical specimens. Comparisons with comparably aged men killed in automobile accidents in the U.S. showed a striking difference: the latter had far less arterial damage. The difference was striking enough to generate a study to try to figure it out.

The search came down to one major difference: the soldiers had to use large quantities of "water-purification tablets" before they could drink any of the water in Vietnam. These tablets were chlorine.

Chlorine is not an innocuous substance. It is a powerful bleaching agent, and it kills bugs. It's highly reactive against living tissue, which is why it works so well to destroy microorganisms, both in our water and on our bathroom tiles. It does not react any less strongly against human tissue, and when ingested, it is carried into the bloodstream, where it can attack the walls of arteries.

The body, on the other hand, in its preprogrammed wisdom, tries to insulate itself from these damaged areas. It does so, apparently, by laying down a tiny layer of cholesterol as a protective coating against these scarred areas.

You can see where we're headed with this. If the scarring continues, the repair efforts continue, until total scarring leads to total "repairing," with arteries then congested with masses of cholesterol. Theoretically, it isn't the cholesterol itself that causes the problem; it's the body's need to use it excessively as a result of abnormal chemical stress.

A positively magnificent, though startling, book on this subject has been written by Joseph M. Price, M.D., who showed in animal studies how fast chlorine in higher doses can do damage and how it never varies. The book is called *Coronaries/Cholesterol/Chlorine*. Dr. Price's simple experiments with chlorine, and his research on the mechanism by which it does its damage, is valuable reading for anyone who is concerned about their health. Though simple, it's an eye opener that can make you think.

If chlorine can kill single-cell organisms (like germs, fungi, etc.), it can also kill multi-cell organisms (you're one of those). It may take awhile, but the effect is there. Avoid it.

Although bromine is less well known, it is in the same chemical class as chlorine. And as far as biological health is concerned, it should not be trusted as an acceptable substitute for water you would want to drink.

Some of the serious pure water advocates respect so strongly what chlorine can do that they advise against even showering or bathing in water treated with it, as the skin, particularly the scalp, is very absorptive. In fact, studies exist directly implying that washing hair in chlorinated water absorbs more of the chemical into the body than is normally ingested through drinking all day!

If that were not enough, imagine compounding the situation by deliberately doing something toxic, something that never had to be done in the first place, and that was not even involved with the purification of water. This runs us into a second danger.

Danger #2

If you look at a list showing all the unwanted chemicals in our water, you would be amazed at its length: tens of thousands of environmental bad guys. The frustrating news is that one of the scariest chemicals is deliberately dumped into our drinking water, and most, though not all, of our water districts are brainwashed enough to allow it. (This applies to the United States only. Nowhere else is this travesty permitted.) More frustrating still is the fact that the issue is so emotionally charged in favor of this chemical, and by people who really do want the best for our health, both our own and our children's.

The number-two bad guy is fluoride. That wonderful stuff that is saving our children from cavities. Let's not waste time here: sodium fluoride is rat poison. Head over to a hardware store and check it out. Most of them still carry it for just that purpose.

I've heard all the arguments from well-meaning, concerned parents who only want the best for their kids. Of course the dose is less than that necessary to kill rats, but our bodies have trouble with the stuff just like rats, and small amounts add up, slowly (or maybe not so slowly) over years. Understand this fact: fluoride is the second most toxic chemical in nature—the only one ranked higher is arsenic (Williams & Wilkins 1984). I'm not making this up.

As a heated topic, this one really sizzles. I ask you to realize that I have no hidden agenda, nothing to sell but this book (and you've already bought that), so if you are in favor of fluoridated water, please hear me out. I am hoping to lead you to known, published information to which you may not have had access. This is a dangerous chemical we're playing with. It was once used therapeutically to depress thyroid activity (Yiamouyiannis 1993). Even if you think we should have small amounts, do you really trust every local utility technician to put only the "right" amount of this poison in your water? (We won't discuss the fact that you weren't asked whether you wanted the stuff in the first place.)

Fluoride is a waste product of aluminum mining. Research concluding that adding fluoride (in amounts higher than you might think) prevented cavities was funded by the aluminum producers. Why not be paid for your waste to be removed for you? (Ah, we have another one of those cute tricks.)

Fluoride is toxic. It is neurotoxic, meaning, in this case, it hits the central nervous system and causes behavioral changes before you get physical findings, like mottling of the teeth—a common side effect. (Mottling is discolored splotches on the front teeth of kids who have gotten too much fluoride; ever seen this?) Dental fluorosis is a disease state stemming from overingestion of this chemical and can start with simple blotches on the teeth and end with loss of affected teeth, in more severe cases.

In 1990, the *New England Journal of Medicine* (March 22 issue) carried a report from the Mayo Clinic stating that a trial of fluoride for osteoporosis caused *increased* hip fractures and bone fragility. Fluoride exposure has been implicated in genetic damage, tumors, and hypersensitivity reactions. Neat stuff, and they put it in our water.

In a report reprinted in the *Health Freedom News,* July, 1995, George Glasser reported that, "Both the Pasteur Institute, France, and the Nobel Institute, Sweden, concur that fluoride has little or no value as a dental cavity deterrent, and stress that the possible health risks from using fluoride outweigh any benefit."

For those with enough of an open mind to look, the definitive answers are already published, thoroughly and unequivocally. Those answers are available from Dr. John Yiamouyiannis, a Ph.D. in biochemistry. His booklet, *Lifesaver's Guide to Fluoridation,* and his full-length book, *Fluoride: The Aging Factor,* are the way to go.

Danger #3

Even after filtration, water often fails to have that crystal-clear look. All the bugs may be dead and all the major particles may be gone, but there still there may be a faint haze. You can't have that . . . people might talk. To avoid this problem, most municipal water supplies apply an additional treatment step that uses aluminum sulfate, commonly called "alum." The idea is that the particulate matter remaining in the water, making it cloudy, forms a complex with the alum and falls out, leaving the water clear.

The problem associated with this is that nobody can guarantee anybody that all the aluminum is gone from the final product. There are those happy to say that most of it is gone, which may be fine for describing the removal of stains from your unmentionables, but we're supposed to drink this stuff.

Aluminum is everywhere. It's in cooking utensils, antiperspirants, snack bags, and every soft drink you can buy. Now it's in the water used to make most of those drinks.

We need minerals. We also need greater or lesser amounts of several metals, but aluminum is not one of them, and like chlorine it definitely is not innocuous. It has been linked to Alzheimer's disease, implicated in premature aging, and is a known biological toxin. It builds up in human tissues, and it's hard to get rid of. You don't need to be drinking the stuff.

The Mineral Danger

I guess this should really be called "The Unmineral Danger," or maybe "The Mineral Situation." In all our efforts to get the smell, taste and color hassle out of "hard" (high-mineral content) water, we missed something: many, if not most, of those minerals are good for us.

Pure water, that is, really pure, 100 percent H_2O is not normal in nature. All water, everywhere, has "impurities." However, these added goodies are predominately minerals, electrolytes, for which the body was designed. Without them, like with pure distilled water, the body has a harder time handling the liquid, apparently, because there is ample evidence that "soft," or mineral-free, water carries a clearly increased risk of cardiovascular disease, including both heart attacks and strokes.

Apparently, the magnesium and calcium salts in harder waters have a considerable protective benefit for our bodies. In fact, I remember, as a child, seeing warnings on bottles of distilled water for steam irons stating that they were not for internal use. The reason certainly was not due to purity; water does not get any purer than by distilling it. I don't think distilled water from time to time is a problem, but it just isn't a healthy solution to our very real city water problem.

This information comes from work starting as far back as the late 1950s, culminating in a published letter in *JAMA* (the official publication of the American Medical Association), by Dr. Andrew Shaper, a member of the United Kingdom Medical Research Council.

The message here is not to throw away your water softener. I just wouldn't drink much of its output. As Dr. Shaper put it, if you have a water softener in use, then leaving one tap in your house disconnected from it, as a source for drinking water, might be regarded as "judicious" (*JAMA*, Vol. 230, No. 1, Oct. 7, 1974). I agree.

Unfortunately (sorry guys), there's more.

Other Dangers

Everything else that can go wrong with water is dumped into this section (kind of like it's dumped into the water). We could go crazy trying to track down the thousands of potential hazards that can end up in our water one way or another. Whether from fertilizers, petrochemicals, industrial wastes, domestic cleaners, acid rain or biological hazards, we will need to deal with them on an overall basis, not one by one. There is just too much out there.

The serious problems have been discussed at enough length to show where I believe the emphasis should lie. You want to avoid anything that Mother Nature did not mean to put into your drinking water (and maybe, occasionally, a few things she did).

So, the idea is to avoid chlorine, fluoride, aluminum, soft (mineral-free) water, disease-causing organisms, and all the other agents that are considered toxic, to the greatest extent possible. "How does one do that?" you ask.

Potential Solutions

On a grander scale (compared to simple home use), the avoidance of chemical processing of water is paramount, as the solution is currently as bad or worse than the problem. The answer, I am convinced, lies in a combination of ultra-violet radiation and ozonation. These modalities are not experimental; they exist now, and are used in many countries that are well advanced in this area and do not consider chlorine an acceptable purifier. (This is almost all of Europe, so we are not talking about pipe dreams. Just keep it in mind if you ever become a politician!)

On the home front, ultraviolet (UV) only and combined UV-ozonating treatment units are available for in-house use. Two good sources of information are: *The Family News*: 800-284-6263; 305-759-8710, www.familyhealthnews.com, and *Ozone News* of the International Ozone Association: 203-348-3542; fax: 203-967-4845; www.int-ozone-assoc.org.

Unfortunately, if you already have "city" water, either it will have to be filtered, to get the chlorine out, or you will have to buy spring water, an expensive long-term proposition. If you try filtration, be careful, because fluoride removal is tough, and most companies avoid telling you what their units will not do, drowning you with all the goodies that they will.

Not all spring waters are alike, and not all bottled waters are spring water. With the increased demand for bottled water, all sorts of qualities are hitting the market. "Drinking" water does not qualify. Your safest bet is to go with a well-known company that draws water from as deep a source as possible and clearly labels their product, including a table of minerals. Search for the milligrams (mg) of magnesium, and find the product with the most you can get.

I don't work for a water company, but I would have to say that Evian™ Spring Water is one of the best for drinking. Check the list of minerals. It is also, unfortunately, the most expensive. In this case I guess you really do get what you pay for.

Water filters, unfortunately, are out there by the dozens, with all sorts of claims and even wider variations in quality. The best very clearly list comparisons of themselves with others, and it does not take long to figure out which lists contain legitimate information. Chlorine removal is vital, and percentage removed is most helpful, along with gallons filtered before needing a filter replacement. There are all types of sizes and capacities. Two places where you can start looking are Multipure Corp: 800-622-9206, 702-360-8880, www.multipure.com and Everpure Corp: 800-942-1153, 630-654-4000, www.everpure.com.

Fluoride is tougher to handle, if you cannot or do not wish to start with water that does not already have it, but still want it gone, then you are probably stuck with a reverse osmosis machine. They are more expensive than straight filters and can mess up some mineral levels. Good spring water is simpler.

Distilled water avoids both fluoride and aluminum, but remember it is entirely devoid of minerals; it is 100 percent pure H_2O, nothing else. This puts you basically in the ultra soft water category, where you may be trading one problem for another. Fill your clothes iron with it, wash in it, but don't drink too much of it.

There probably is no ideal solution. You will just have to take the parameters of your given situation, evaluate how scared you are by the situation, then decide how far you are willing to go. Anything you do has to be better than leaving your head in the sand . . . or in the water.

CHAPTER 5

Artificial vs. Natural

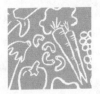

EVERYWHERE YOU LOOK, on almost every food label (and therefore in almost every food), there are multitudes of artificial substances and processes—colors, flavors, preservatives, "enhancers," emulsifiers, fortifiers, purifiers, and so forth—not to mention homogenization, pasteurization and irradiation. The list is almost endless, with many of the items not even pronounceable, much less understandable. Some things they don't even tell you about, like residual pesticides, synthetic hormones, artificial fertilizers, or even gases to make unripe foods artificially ripen.

Is there a problem with all these nonfood items and procedures in what is supposed to just be food? Does "better living through chemistry" really apply to what we eat?

Food Additives

Consider the purposes of many of these agents: preservatives, for example, are for shelf life, not your life. The colors are purely cosmetic, which can only relate to the food's visual desirability, while flavors and flavor enhancers are for palatability, implying that the food itself, for some reason, doesn't taste that great without them. The convenience provided by antifoaming, anticaking, or emulsifying agents (imagine having to actually stir the stuff ourselves) is difficult to ignore.

What also seems hard to ignore, however, is that nearly all these functions are for purely marketing, not nutritional, purposes; so some degree of care should be taken before blindly gobbling down the contents of a wrapper listing a bunch of mystery ingredients on the label. Just because "when it rains, it pours," that does not mean it's the best for you. Time and time again these "wonder" chemicals and processes are shown to carry the price of having undesirable side effects, due to the fact that the body was never designed for their assimilation. Even scarier is the fact that often these ill effects are not immediate, sometimes taking years, or even decades, for the consequences to become known.

Food Substitutes

Besides food additives, what about food substitutes? There's no beating around the bush here; we're replacing the entire thing with something that is, by definition, a counterfeit. Why? What was wrong with the original? Is margarine better than butter? Is coffee creamer better than cream? Is "processed cheese product" better than cheese? Are artificial sweeteners generally better than sugar?

Let's bypass the media hype, the Madison Avenue brainwashing, and really take a look at what has happened to what we eat and why. It's important. There are two general areas to consider:

1. Real foods that have been adulterated by either artificial processes or synthetic chemicals.
2. Totally synthetic, artificial "foods."

Artificial Processes

There are several processes that, in my opinion, change real foods into an artificial state. This area would potentially be the most controversial one because we could argue over the point at which one considers a food changed enough to be called artificial.

An example of this type of perversion of our food supply would be the homogenization of peanut butter. This much-loved food, if naturally ground and allowed to sit, will settle into two layers, leaving oil at the top and concentrated "peanut stuff" underneath. It's a bit of a chore to stir the layers back together, so food processing companies, in their ultimate wisdom, simplify things for us by "homogenizing" the product into a state that will not separate by itself. You don't even have to refrigerate it! (We'll leave the discussion of rancidity of foods left at room temperature for another time.)

Milk is treated the same way. When homogenized, the cream molecules are chopped up so fine that they will not settle out, so the liquid no longer needs to be shaken. (It also can no longer have the cream poured off at home like years ago.) There is also the possibility, unfortunately, that the process has some deleterious side effects, stemming from the breaking up of large molecules into smaller ones, allowing the absorption of substances through the gut wall that previously were too big to cross.

What pasteurization does to foods is a bit too controversial to consider here, but irradiation of foods, like milk, obviously makes changes that were not intended by nature. "Milk" that can sit on a shelf at room temperature for months to years just cannot be the same stuff the cow started with. (Even the bugs won't touch it!) The destruction of major amounts of nutrients, not just bacteria, is beyond question. How much destruction does it take before deficiencies set in?

Consider bread or, more generically, flour. This magnificent staple food has sustained man for thousands of years. The grain family truly can be the "staff of life," but beware. Almost all (and I mean very nearly all) the breads, rolls, muffins, cakes, pies, cookies, etc. that are available to us today are anything but natural. As you'll recall from Chapter 3, any flour that is white, wheat, bleached or even enriched, has been processed and refined, so the nutrients required for the body's utilization of that flour (and therefore its nutrient density) are almost entirely gone. Don't forget our glorious "enrichment" process, artificially adding back a few synthetic vitamins, like robbing someone of all their new clothes and giving them back an old pair of tennis shoes. Even the grain's own fiber, needed to slow the breakdown of the flour's starch (to sugar!), is removed.

All these changes serve to create an artificial food, which is an oxymoron (neat word, and well worth looking up). There is always something missing in the changed state, something that we needed to fully absorb and utilize the food item for our own nourishment.

And what do we gain? Quite simply, a more marketable item. In the case of flour, it is a lighter color, has a lighter weight, a smoother texture or, most importantly, an increased shelf life. Don't kid yourself; you should know by now that very few of these unnatural changes to our food are for your health.

Synthetic Chemicals

Look at the foods that are adulterated by chemicals instead of processes. (Of course, many foods, in one way or another, are both.) Nearly all the commercial food colors are artificial, meaning they have nothing to do with nourishment . . . absolutely nothing. When you see "F, D & C #" on the label, it stands for a dye, nothing more than a paint to make a "food" (or whatever) look more appealing, period.

This philosophy also includes chemicals that have no color themselves, but keep a food looking fresh when in reality it's not. (Wouldn't you want to know when a food is artificially held in a fresh-looking state, when in fact it's not?) This allows food to continue to look fresh and be sold to you when it would otherwise look so bad that you would never consider putting it in your mouth. Some of the common bad guys are nitrates, nitrites, sulfites, bisulfites and sulfur dioxide.

Have you ever seen restaurants with signs on their salad bars that say, "Bisulfites added," or something similar? (Look for them;

these signs are not at all uncommon, but they are not particularly prominent, either.) Commercial establishments have used the chemicals for years, long before they started advertising the fact. Was it an attack of conscience that they now bother to tell you?

Not at all. In fact, enough people have had serious (including fatal) allergic reactions to these agents that a user must now tell you when they are being used. Fortunately, a sort of reversal has begun—some restaurants now brag about the fact that they do not use these chemicals, the purpose of which was never anything other than what to me constitutes a fraud dumped on a hungry public.

To play it safe, assume both artificial flavors and flavor enhancers are purely non-nutritive chemical additives for palatability, put in solely to make you either eat something—or possibly to make you eat more of it (pleasant thought). The "betcha can't eat just one" philosophy is not aimed at your health or your ideal weight; it's aimed at your wallet, which is the only place you end up lighter.

The most notorious and most pervasive flavor enhancer is monosodium glutamate (MSG). This stuff is everywhere and avoiding it takes some real work. Many people have allergic reactions to it, so once they track down the cause, they know more quickly what's going on. The rest of us aren't so lucky.

The "chemicalized" foods are not just flavored and colored. The number of agents available to change your food to an unnatural state is in the many thousands. Really. Often, when the purpose is not for perverting your concept of proper flavor or color, it's for enhancing the convenience of the food manufacturer (an appropriate word). That is, the chemical is added to keep the food from gumming up the processing machine, separating out, spoiling too soon, or some such thing.

Even the addition of vitamins is more to make the item appealing than to really augment your health. The amounts added are tiny; the vitamins are cheap synthetic ones; and the number used, compared to all those now available, is ridiculously small, in most cases.

The list of chemicals added to our foods is growing longer, not shorter. Each year, food conventions offer new and more diversified means of doing things to our foodstuffs to make them more convenient, last longer, smell better or taste better; but almost never is the effort just to make foods better for us. Until we realize that fact and cause the marketplace to change its supply based on our change in demand, we will continue to be inundated by these artificial foods and food additives.

Read labels—and read them carefully. Pick up a technical dictionary, and find out what you are putting in your mouth and what its purpose is. When you hit a big list of words you cannot pronounce, be careful . . . you are most likely playing "the artificial game," and it's one that is better left unplayed, because the consumer rarely wins.

Synthetic Foods

Now, what about food substitutes, completely artificial, synthetic "stuff to eat," compared to real food?

To me, this is where it gets a bit bizarre because I can't really picture anyone actually entertaining the thought that something totally artificial could be anything but totally disastrous as food.

Take margarine, for example. Compared to butter (which can also have artificial additives), margarine is, quite simply, manufactured, plastic butter. Since the mid 1970s, studies have consistently shown that the artificial fats (trans fatty acids), formed during the process of bubbling hydrogen gas through liquid oils to produce margarine, cause considerable trouble in the human body.

If it were not for a brilliant advertising campaign by those who stand to make a bundle by selling such second-rate stuff, nobody would ever dream of actually buying it. The problem is that margarine is so cheap to make that it is well worth the effort to dupe us into eating it.

By the way, don't kid yourself. If something gets into the body that the body cannot handle, then some kind of damage, somewhere, is occurring. It's happened time and time again. The problem is it always takes too long for us to actually see the damage to make the association with what caused it. If you got sick two minutes after eating something artificial, you would never eat it again and that would be that.

Powdered nondairy coffee creamers—here's something that hasn't been within 100 miles of a cow or any other living thing, yet we pump it into our bodies by the ton when we're told how "fresh" it tastes. Drinking coffee, black or otherwise, is one issue, but this is ridiculous.

Artificial sweeteners are unabashedly presented to us as totally synthetic manufactured chemicals. Comparing these to sugar is a bit tougher than it looks, which is why Chapter 2 was devoted to a large part of the issue. Obviously, I believe natural is almost exclusively superior to artificial. The problem is, today's "pure cane sugar" is basically artificial, too, being nothing like the original sugar cane. It's a pure chemical, maybe even a drug. Once it has been processed, refined, and concentrated, with all the vitamins, minerals, and fiber required for its assimilation removed, it is much more difficult to say whether sugar is better than today's blatantly artificial sweeteners. (At least the synthetic ones are a bit more honest.)

As I've said, there may be occasional advantages to some of the synthetic sweeteners, if truly natural sugars are unavailable, and you just must have something sweet. I trust aspartame™ the least, due to voluminous reports of problems with the drug, as reported to the U.S. Food & Drug Administration (FDA). It's a minor shame that a less toxic artificial sweetener, Sucaryl™, is available in Canada, Mexico, and worldwide, but blacklisted in the U.S. due to some fast "research" work by sugar interests.

If you must eat something sweet, however, the more nutrient density the better, though it may take more searching to find dehydrated date crystals, totally raw dark honey, or other natural sweeteners, including the hard-to-find stevia. Use the least amount possible, of course, and read labels carefully.

How about artificial bread? This was a media blitz for awhile, but has cooled down a bit. The "bread" has a synthetic starch in it that the body cannot use; therefore, you get the feel of having eaten bread without any of the starch breakdown to sugar, and hence no calories. And probably no other nutrients.

Of course, there's the one we've all been waiting for (well, not all): artificial fat! Approved by the FDA, it's called olestra, or the brand name Olean™. More neat stuff. You don't absorb calories from this fat, but you also don't get the fat-soluble vitamins. (It's okay, they throw in only a few.) Since we're told that's not a problem, all you have to worry about is abdominal cramping, loose stools, and (best of all) the dreaded "anal leak." In the words of Alan Gaby, M.D., "Because it is a nonabsorbable oily material, olestra has the potential to slip unnoticed past the anal sphincter, producing an embarrassing oil stain on one's clothing" (Gaby 1996). Marvelous.

The Point

Humanity has existed on this planet for a long time—just how long depends on your religious or scientific convictions, but regardless, it's a really long time. In all those past millenia man has only had natural foods. Though we may have cooked it, salted it, and a few other things, it remained whole, natural food for thousands of years. In all that time the systems of our bodies have never had any contact with the totally alien molecules present in what we now loosely label as "food." That's a really bad deal.

Biological organisms can get used to many things, similar to how bacteria can become more tolerant to, and then survive, large amounts of antibiotics that once would have killed them in minute doses. (We'll get to some of that in the next chapter.) However, full organ systems in creatures of the sophistication of human beings require huge amounts of time, some even say millions of years, to acclimate to totally new chemical structures. Most of the new ones we're dealing with from our food industry have been around only in the last few decades. The food/chemical combines are not sleeping. There are new "miracle foods" coming out all the time. The very latest as of this writing is a new release by the FDA of a huge volume of "genetically engineered" foods. These are goodies with spliced genes from lots of different sources incorporated into their original structure, all predominantly for increased shelf life.

Maybe these new "advances" will save the world, ending cancer, making us all skinny, with no risk of heart disease. Maybe not.

The question of artificial versus natural at times can be a heated controversy, especially with the food conglomerates controlling some major purse strings. The rule I recommend, however, is this: If man messed with it, don't eat it.

A Nutritional Insurance Policy

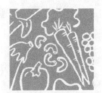

CHAPTER 6

Protecting the Gut

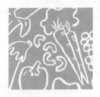

THE GASTROINTESTINAL (GI) TRACT, or "gut," is where nearly all absorption of nutrients takes place. We can design a magnificent (and potentially expensive) nutrient regimen for achieving optimal health, but if it isn't absorbed, it'll just pass right through. What a waste (literally). I have no problem with "expensive urine" (there are some good reasons to strive for that), but there's absolutely no need for expensive stool. We'll be dealing with proper digestion in chapter 11, and adding a few more ideas concerning proper gut function in chapter 16, but our nutritional insurance policy needs to be underwritten with a knowledge of the simple little single-cell friends that we very much need inhabiting our GI tract. With that in mind, we also need to be aware of the role antibiotics can play in disturbing this most sensitive environment.

Beware the Trusty Antibiotic

I remember, as a new physician just starting out in an outpatient clinic in Jacksonville, Florida, the first episodes of the flu to hit the area that year. Our office was rural at the time, and there were many older "country" types of patients, very set in their ways. They would come in and, more times than I care to remember, say something to the tune of "Well, Doc, here I am with the flu again, so I need my antibiotic."

Believe it or not, most of them actually said "my" antibiotic, that lifesaving drug that brought them back from an achy, feverish brink of death so many times before.

With symptoms consistent with the flu, I spent considerable time and effort explaining that the flu does not respond to antibiotics—not even a little bit—any more than the common cold does, since both illnesses are caused by viruses, not bacteria. The patient would then leave with medications for symptomatic relief, to wait out the next few days until the discomfort subsided, and things were back to normal. Or so I thought.

I'd move ahead to the next appointment, smugly satisfied that I'd done my best for the patient. Meanwhile, the patient has headed across the street, literally, to obtain the life-giving antibiotic that has saved him in the past. More than once, I discovered, clients would pay for a second office visit, with another physician, just to get the antibiotic they felt they needed. (Not to mention, of course, the fact that they never would come back!). I was learning.

In modern medicine this event is not really all that uncommon. It's not uncommon because of a belief system that seems so logical. This belief is so common, in fact, and so logical, that I give its existence a name. I call it the "Conventional Illness Progression":

You get sick → *You take an antibiotic* → *You get better*

It's so logical, so simple. Everyone knows antibiotics are lifesaving, maybe even good for you as a preventive. They aren't even on prescription in Mexico—anyone can get one, anytime.

It's so logical that many people have never even considered trying the progression an even simpler way: without the middle part.

So what's the problem? Is this just much ado about nothing? Is it really that big a deal to take an antibiotic now and then?

Much Ado About Nothing?

Let's get one thing straight: Antibiotics are unquestionably, as a class, responsible for saving more lives than any other drug type. They are truly "miracle drugs." (In my opinion maybe the *only* miracle drugs.) At its advent, half a century ago, penicillin, when administered to patients unquestionably doomed to die of pneumonia, caused them to practically, if not literally, leap out of their deathbeds. This is after taking what today is considered an incredibly low dose of the drug. Similar histories abound worldwide. More antibiotics, of all levels of toxicity, were then designed, and the drug company races were on, with profits at stake that none of us can in any way really fathom. (From this start came the "miracle drug" fixation: If a drug can save the life of a loved one, sometimes in as little as a few hours, think of the things that are possible with new patent medicines! But I digress.)

Don't misunderstand; antibiotics have done phenomenal things for us, and when truly necessary, they may be the only difference between life and death, in certain circumstances.

We all know the upside; let's examine the downside.

The Downside of Antibiotics

Anyone who has ever had an antibiotic prescribed has probably been told to "take all of it," and most people know that it is because there is the distinct possibility of teaching bacteria to become "antibiotic resistant." In this situation, the strongest bugs die last, and if they are not totally eradicated, the survivors can pass on to future populations the genetic information required to survive subsequent onslaughts of the drug. This is precisely why original doses of penicillin, years ago, were given in the neighborhood of 100,000 units, while today many millions of units are required for the same bug, if the antibiotic works at all. (Some bugs even learn to feed on the antibiotic!)

This is one reason for the plethora of new antibacterials, in addition to the profit motive. The same bugs just aren't dying the way they used to. (Plus, of course, some bugs did not respond to penicillin in the first place.) Unfortunately, many of these newer drugs do not have the safety record that penicillin has built up for itself. Except for relatively rare allergic reactions, which can be rapidly fatal, penicillin is remarkably safe in extremely high doses. Many other antibiotics, however, have mildly severe, to truly serious side effects and toxicities.

So, there is an increasing amount of drug resistance, an increasing number of antibacterial drugs which are themselves toxic, plus allergic reactions (which may themselves be on the increase). This situation, by itself, makes antibiotics a double-edged sword, to be respected at least enough not to hand them out to every sniffle that comes in the door.

However, none of this is the cause of the chronic problem that I fear is the really sinister downside of today's antibiotics.

Antibiotics are nonselective. I don't mean, of course, that they kill everything, or we'd only need one drug, so they must be somewhat selective. The problem is, this selection isn't restricted to the invading, disease-causing bugs. The message here is, almost without exception (in fact, the only exception I can think of is a relatively very small class called the antifungal agents), all antibiotics kill "good guys" as well as "bad guys."

This is obviously a survivable phenomenon, or we would all be dead. The human body is loaded with beneficial bacteria, basically throughout the entire digestive tract (the mouth, throat, esophagus, stomach, small intestine, large intestine, rectum). These bacteria are considered "good guys" because they serve a beneficial purpose in the digestion and assimilation of our foods. They are not parasitic—they are synergistic, meaning that they help us out, and in return we supply them with a home.

There are, of course, all sorts of bacteria that are considered normal inhabitants of the digestive tract. *E. coli* is present in the colon and under certain circumstances can be the cause of disease, especially in the urinary tract. The real "good guys," however, are bacteria like *Lactobacillus acidophilus* (*L. acidophilus*), and *L. bifidus*. These forms are instrumental in aiding our digestion and serve no known ill purpose. We get a dose of them as we come through the birth canal (mouth open and face first, usually), since they are also normal inhabitants of a woman's vaginal tract. (The only difference is that *L. acidophilus* has a different name, in the vagina, where it is called Doderlein's bacilli.)

The fact that we are not immediately killed by antibiotics does not mean there is no danger here. The synergistic bacteria may take awhile to be killed off to the extent that we even show any symptoms, much less to the point that we might be in some serious jeopardy. However, the jeopardy is still there, for a simple reason: When compared to the invading or disease-causing organisms, the good guys die first.

This is a biggie, so please don't underestimate what is going on here. The beneficial germs are not as well "trained" as the invading organisms in the art of warfare. Genetically, their abilities do not include invading and forcing a place for themselves, as do many of the pathogenic (disease-causing) ones. The invaders often will get a toehold in an area where the body's immune defenses have weakened. While the benevolent types are not nearly so aggressive as the invaders—the slightest disruption and the beneficial germs are weakened or even finished off completely. (The cliché "nice guys finish last" certainly seems to be true in the germ world! And it's a race of some real significance.)

So What?

When this happens, a sequence of events is initiated that can lead to chronic illness if not deliberately interrupted. Women especially are aware of an early stage of this when, after taking an antibiotic (for almost any cause), they may experience a vaginal yeast "infection." This uncomfortable disease is nothing more than the lowering of the defenses in the vagina by killing off Doderlein's bacilli. Once these bacteria are gone, the yeast have no competition in the neighborhood, so they move in. (Like viruses, yeasts are not at all bothered by antibiotics.)

The predominant troublemaker is called *Candida albicans*, a common yeast that is basically everywhere but does not cause trouble as long as the body's defenses are up to snuff. Unfortunately, antibiotics are not the only drug class to cause problems. Steroids, birth-control pills, and other hormones can contribute, but antibiotics are the worst, since they directly kill bacteria.

Remember, though, this killing effect is nonselective. When a woman takes an antibiotic for, say, a sinus infection, the drug does not merely kill bad bugs in the sinuses; it simultaneously decides to go kill friendly bacteria in the vagina. The vaginal bacteria, or flora, are the same ones that are in the digestive tract. So, while symptoms are showing up in one area (yeast in the vagina), changes are starting in the other (altered flora in the gut), even if symptoms have not yet occurred. Benevolent flora are dying anywhere they exist, affected by a drug that is carried anywhere that blood flows (and it flows a lot of places).

The symptoms may even already be present: variable diarrhea of no known cause, constipation, cramping, gas, "indigestion," food intolerances, slow stomach emptying, abdominal pain, and others, though we might not attach importance to them. Instead, we take an antacid, a laxative, or whatever, from the over-the-counter armamentarium of drugs that exists for those purposes. Don't bother thinking of a cause; it's part of a "high-stress" existence, and treating symptoms is all we can do about it. *Don't believe it.*

Obviously, I am not saying that all symptoms are caused by killing off the flora in the gut. However, I am saying that if you are chronically troubled with more than one of the above problems, and you have a history of multiple courses of antibiotics, then you might consider altered gut flora as a highly contributing factor. What's really neat here is that if you treat yourself as if this is, in fact, the cause, and you are wrong, you have done no harm to yourself. That is why it's worth considering.

How about your kids? Have they had lots of ear infections, usually treated with antibiotics? (Maybe the drugs were necessary, but I sure would look for food allergies if the problem is recurrent.) As a caring parent, have you taken your child to the doctor for every sniffle? Bear in mind, when you go to the doctor, he is placed in the position of having to actually do something, otherwise he may appear unconcerned. Why not play it safe and just give an antibiotic? Many parents are programmed to be upset if they do not get one, through no fault of their own, while doctors are forced to "cover" themselves and give one, through no fault of their own. (There is always the possibility of a bacterial infection coming—or lawsuit.)

Ever see a white, pasty covering on your child's tongue (that won't scrape off)? That is most likely thrush, by definition a yeast infection of the tongue. I don't believe it's possible to have thrush without yeast farther down the digestive tract. This finding is becoming increasingly common in infants (where it is expected), and I have seen it many times in high school teenagers (where it isn't). I believe this trend is caused by a combination of our excessively high dietary sugar intake (bacteria feed on sugar) and antibiotics. (See Chapter 2.)

In medical school, I was taught that antibiotics could do things similar to what I have described, but I was never told what to do about it. We weren't even told to worry, unless it reached serious proportions, when you might have to give another antibiotic to fix the problem caused by a specific bacterial takeover from a resistant bug!

What to Do

Obviously, it is desirable to use antibiotics as little as possible. Depending on the circumstances, however, this may or may not be all that easy to do. The real issue is what to do if you think symptoms are already present that may be caused by systemic yeast.

Much of the solution exists over the counter and has for centuries, though now stronger versions are available. We are right back to our friend, *L. acidophilus*, for a start. European women have long known that plain yogurt, directly applied to the vagina, is not only soothing, but also usually curative for yeast infections by replacing the "competition" and fighting the yeast. Today's standard solution is nearly always to kill off the bad guys without ever replacing the good ones. This is obviously only half a solution (and, in some cases, not even that), which is why some women are haunted by recurrences. Remember also that we have still done nothing for the gut, which may very well be simultaneously affected.

Eating yogurt is a major step toward normalization, but it has to be real yogurt with active cultures, so that the acidophilus cultures are still alive. It also should be plain flavor, since sugar is something that *Candida albicans* feeds strongly on. Plain yogurt, however, is not particularly palatable to most, and it also is not very strong as a source of cultures. Fortunately, there is an option better than yogurt.

Actually, *L. acidophilus* is available directly, and in much stronger concentrations than yogurt. It can be obtained as a powder, capsule, or liquid, but I recommend the powder due to the fact that it coats immediately, unlike a capsule, and tastes better than the liquid. Also, it can be purchased in a nondairy form, necessary for many. Get the strongest doses possible, which are the billions of "colony-forming units," (CFU), or sometimes just "units."

Such supplements often are mixed with other forms of beneficial bacterial cultures, which is fine, and there are controversies over which tolerate stomach acid the best. There are many excellent products out there. Some trial and error may be needed to find the best for you, as rarely there can be mild allergic reactions to high doses. These are taken with meals, so they are better distributed, but if you have indigestion symptoms, they can be taken anytime and often offer considerable relief without side effects.

Besides avoiding sugar, one must cut down on high-yeast foods as much as possible in the beginning of treatment to lessen the initial stress load of the body with yeast. This means avoiding things like mushrooms, brewer's yeast, leavened breads, moldy foods, beer, wine, and refined flour, which quickly converts to sugar in the body. If symptoms subside after treatment, then through experimentation one may begin reintroducing desired foods to see which are tolerated.

A superb book on this subject is *The Yeast Connection Handbook* by William Crook, M.D., and I highly recommend this reference if you, or someone you know, may have this problem or a history that may put you in jeopardy of manifesting it later.

So far, the body's stress load from yeast has been lessened, and we have tried to re-establish the acidophilus, but nothing yet has been done to actually kill the fungus. There are now over-the-counter drugs for vaginal yeast, but none for oral use. In the health food store, however, there are herbal and other compounds for this purpose. The most popular is caprylic acid, which, in many people, is very effective. Also, garlic extract (Kwai™, Kyolic™, Garlicin™, and Nu Pro™ for example) is another way to make the environment hostile for yeast. More recently, olive leaf extract and grapefruit seed extract have become popular.

It is possible that stronger antifungal agents may be necessary, which unfortunately means that you are restricted to the consideration of prescription drugs, such as nystatin powder (Nilstat™), ketoconazole (Nizoral™), and fluconazole (Diflucan™). Nystatin, as a liquid, is weaker, and contains both sugar and dye. The powder form is a better selection, even over pills, but it is harder to find a pharmacist that carries it.

Conclusion

Antibiotics, when necessary, are magnificent drugs. The important thing to keep in mind, however, is that they are very much a double-edged sword and need to be respected as such. As opposed to being innocuous, they can carry considerable and long-lasting effects, besides just short-term side effects. They are not vitamins and should not be treated as such.

Before you demand your next antibiotic from your doctor, ask his opinion about whether he really thinks it is necessary, or ask whether the problem could be viral, allergic or something else. There is nearly always time to start the drug later, and when there is not time, usually the symptoms tell the doctor right away. At that point, he would not give you a choice.

Too often, when one has the flu or something similar, the progression of "have illness, need antibiotic, get better," also fits the progression of "have illness, get better." Many people just have never tried it that way.

The Appendix includes book recommendations for alternatives

to different types of medications. Keep reading and get informed. Be sure you need that antibiotic. If you need it, by all means take it. Just be aware of the possible consequences, and consider at least a short addendum of acidophilus to your long-term nutritional insurance policy.

CHAPTER 7

You Don't Need to Take Vitamins If . . .

WE'VE ALL HEARD IT: "You don't need to take vitamins." Maybe you've heard, "You get all the vitamins you need in the food you eat," or "They'll just give you expensive urine," or "Just eat a balanced diet" or something to that effect. From time to time you may even hear the scary stuff, "Vitamins are dangerous," or "More than the RDA (Recommended Daily Allowance) is toxic." My favorite is the expensive urine one—it's kind of catchy.

It's hard not to be too sarcastic because this subject has been a frustrating one for me for years. There is a deluge of so-called experts, even in medical school (*especially* in medical school), ready at a moment's notice to discuss, at length, the useless waste of time and money invested in taking vitamins and other supplements. Then, of course, there's the inherent toxicity danger, of vitamins of course—not drugs. They love the cute, condescending remarks, often with minimal substance . . . or worse.

It's my turn, so permit me a little sarcasm. For the time being, let's assume you eat a "balanced diet"; you don't eat a lot of "junk food," you exercise moderately from time to time, and you watch your fat and cholesterol. Do you need to take vitamin supplements? It's possible that you don't. But, just how possible is it?

A lot of experts, or at least those said to be experts (or possibly those who should be experts), including the American Medical Association, many family doctors, TV hotshots, etc., continually inundate us with warnings about wasting money on useless pills, quack remedies and health store ripoffs. Could they be right? It's possible that they are. But not very. To really determine our own needs, we need to establish not only what, but also who we're discussing. The fact that we are, of course, discussing you, is more significant than it sounds. In the U.S. (by law), foods, supplements, condiments, anything we eat, must display information on the label concerning nutrient content. Previously the data was in percentages of the Recommended Daily Allowances (RDA) for that item. Of course, only a few nutrients were listed, but you would find them on every food label of the outer packaging. Now it's the "percent daily value" (percent DV), which is even less significant and provides even less information.

The problem is, none of those labels is talking about you. It's not splitting hairs to say that you have nothing to do with what in a laboratory is designated as the average person. Realistically we aren't interested in the theoretically "average" person for whom all those RDAs/DVs are designed. We are interested in an individual—you or someone you care about—not a crash-test dummy that's supposed to be "average," the American standard. The significance of this is monumental because no two people on the planet are alike, not even identical twins. Our biochemical individuality dictates that we may need to build some leeway for the individual differences into our nutritional plan.

The RDAs don't do that. What's worse, the RDAs do not even recognize many of the nutrients that have since been discovered and independently shown to be important, which affect a myriad of our body functions. If each person is different, can anyone design a single requirement list for us all? If it's possible at all, is there a list that is superior to the RDA list? We'll get to that, but the real question, for a beginner, is even more basic: Do you or your loved ones each get all that is needed in the diet without taking nutritional supplements? The answer, hopefully, lies in a series of "ifs" (see sidebar).

You Don't Need Nutritional Supplements If . . .

1. IF you are not living in a high-stress environment, physically or emotionally.
2. IF you easily handle those stresses that do occur.
3. IF you never drink chlorinated water. (Chlorine is a highly reactive molecule—that's how it kills microorganisms.) Fluoridated, chlorinated water is even worse (remember fluoride is rat poison—really!).
4. IF you do not breathe polluted air. (Only very recently has the presence of "free radicals" and the damage caused to our bodies by them been recognized by the same powers that have established, but not changed, our decades old nutritional requirements.)
5. IF you regularly get adequate sleep. (Major amounts of bodily repair occur while we are asleep, when the body can shut down or minimize the activity of processes required for us to function adequately at the conscious level.)
6. IF you do not need over-the-counter medicines for complaints like headache, cough, sore throat, insomnia, indigestion, heartburn, stuffy nose, constipation, etc. (Almost universally these items are toxic . . . read the label warnings. The body was not designed for these agents, and internal organ systems must remove them. This translates directly into states of chemical stress, where those organs must do a job that was never in their union contract.)
7. IF your food is eaten fresh, either raw, steamed, or quick-fried in a wok. (Most foods lose significant vitamins and enzymes within one hour of harvesting or opening.)
8. IF your food is harvested ripe—not early so it ships better.
9. IF your food is not gassed, colored, or coated to look better.
10. IF your food has never been sprayed with toxic pesticides.
11. IF your food has never been stimulated in its growth by synthetic fertilizers (almost all commercially available, grown foods are treated this way, instead of natural compost with full-spectrum nutrients).

12. IF your food has never been stimulated with hormones. (The meat and milk we eat still contain traces of those hormones. Aren't our kids hitting puberty earlier now?)

13. IF your food has no artificial additives for flavor, texture, aroma or shelf-life (not your life). (If they are artificial, these additives must be removed by a human body that considers them toxic because it was not designed for such alien molecules. Our body is a marvel at removing most of them, but there is still a biochemical price.)

14. IF your food has no processed oils on it or in it. (Good luck—almost all oils today are processed.)

15. IF your baked foods have no hydrogenated oils aboard (check the labels. Hydrogenation is a totally synthetic process that forms a type of fatty acid [trans-type] that our bodies are not equipped to handle.)

16. IF your dairy foods are certified raw, so all enzymes are intact. (Real milk [i.e., raw] is much maligned for a multitude of reasons we cannot cover here.)

17. IF your milk is not homogenized, so the reactive molecule xanthine oxidase cannot be broken up and reach the bloodstream. (Pasteurized, homogenized [but vitamin D enriched!] milk is not fit for human consumption, in my opinion. It even makes cows sick, for Pete's sake! For superb information on the subject, I strongly recommend the book *The Milk Book*, by William C. Douglass, M.D. If you are a heavy milk drinker, this fun book is worth your while.)

18. IF your salts have all their original minerals intact. (Even high-priced sea salts are almost devoid of them. Minerals are worth far too much sold separately to give them to you.)

19. IF you eat no refined sugar in your diet. (In America?! I'm afraid the verdict is guilty for me on this one. As a confirmed "sugar-holic," I try to be good, but how can you avoid it all?

20. IF you eat no refined flour in your breads. (Real, whole-grain bread exists, but it's hard to find.)

21. IF you eat no refined flour in your pasta. (Do you eat only whole-wheat, artichoke, spinach, or brown-rice pasta?)

22. IF you eat only whole grains. (brown rice, hulled barley, etc.)
23. IF you eat slowly and chew thoroughly. (This is not a small one. Established medicine never addresses the subject of proper digestion and subsequent absorption of necessary nutrients. Fast eaters pay a price here.)
24. IF you don't overeat.
25. IF you eat multiple, small meals, instead of a few large ones. (This is more of the digestion/absorption issue.)
26. IF your body produces all the digestive enzymes it needs for optimum digestion and absorption of all classes of foods (fat, protein, carbohydrate, including specific sugars like lactose, etc.)
27. IF you rarely mix sugars and proteins at the same meal, since different acid levels are needed in the stomach for proper digestion of each. (What does this say about the "balanced diet"? Try separating these items at two meals and see if you think digestion is faster and more comfortable that way.)
28. IF your gastric (stomach) acid levels are sufficient for breakdown of well-chewed food. (These levels tend to decrease as we age.)
29. IF your insulin is produced and secreted in the right amounts at the right times to properly handle sugar intake.
30. IF your gall bladder works right. (If, in fact, it's still there.)
31. IF all your enzyme systems (thousands of them) work properly in the absorption of nutrients, production of energy, repair of all sorts of damage, and general body maintenance.
32. IF you have not had multiple courses of antibiotics over the years. (This is an underrated danger, as beneficial bacteria are quickly destroyed as our body tries kill invading organisms that have better abilities to defend themselves against the ever-growing arsenal of antibiotics at our disposal.

    Those pharmaceutical companies can really crank them out. We may need them, but it is a double-edged sword and a biochemical stress.)
33. IF you have not taken hormones, including cortisone, pred-

nisone, or birth control pills (difficult for women to avoid at one time or another).

34. IF you have not needed major surgery, a big physical stress.
35. IF you have inherited a perfect immune system from your parents.
36. IF there are no genetic deficiencies in your inherited make up.
37. IF you don't smoke (and never have).
38. IF you only drink very moderately or not at all.
39. IF you rotate the foods in your diet regularly.
40. IF I'm not boring you.

If all, or even most, of the "ifs" in the accompanying sidebar apply to you, then you can safely assume that you do not need nutritional supplements, and your urine would be, in fact, too expensive after all.

If most of these "ifs" apply to you, then you can safely assume that you do not need nutritional supplements. Bear in mind, this list is only partially tongue in cheek: the "If's" are real stresses which, though meant to make a point through their monotony, are factors with which most of us constantly deal in our daily lives.

Once the fallacy of a single RDA for everyone becomes apparent, the next eye opener is to realize that all of these government allowances, besides being outdated, are generated to avoid *deficiencies only*. They do not allow for the possibility of enhanced or optimal nutritional states from doses above those necessary merely to keep you from openly showing a true deficiency, like scurvy, beriberi or rickets. In my opinion, there's a lot more to be had out of life, and at least a little of it, nowadays, must come from a supplement bottle.

Nothing works for everyone, but most people feel better. Placebo effect? Power of suggestion? Maybe. If nothing else, we're talking insurance here.

Although some of the "ifs" apply to me, not enough do. My genetic make-up has its problems, and I eat sugar from time to time. We all breathe the same air. However, I do take nutritional supplements and lots of them. (As an M.D. vitamin taker, that makes me a bit unusual, but hopefully this is becoming less rare.)

Obviously, I do not believe it's possible for anyone living in the United States to get what they need nutritionally just by consuming the food they have at their disposal. Nearly everything in our environment is different (i.e., worse) than it was years ago, from the air and water to the quality of the foods presented to us. Many don't qualify as food at all. When you add in the stresses, both chemical and environmental, coming at us from all directions today, I just don't see how anyone with an open mind can ignore the need for the "insurance policy" of nutritional supplements.

Where Do You Go from Here?

So, where do you go from here? Assuming you want to take some vitamins, how should you begin? Health food stores and vitamin catalogs carry a positively bewildering array of supplements from which to choose. Is there a rational way for a beginner to start? (We're going to discuss this in more detail later in the book, but now is a good time for a brief introduction.)

Supplements are like a football team: You have to put a full team on the playing field before worrying about improving individual players. Buying the latest fad nutrient by itself is not the answer. The greatest quarterback on the planet could not beat a junior high school football team by himself. This concept allows us to cut the "pill field" down to the multivitamin preparations—of which there are still plenty of "teams." My biases for cutting the decision down even further are as follows:

• Avoid hard pills. Some of them are so tightly packed that your digestive system may be unable to break them down. Believe it or not, I have had patients actually report that their supplements have been spotted, unchanged, in their stool. (I have never had the nerve to find out just how that observation has been made.) Anyway, there are too many malabsorptive people in this world to take a chance. This narrows the field to multivitamins in capsule, liquid and powder forms.
• Avoid time-release preparations, which are specifically designed

to only give up the nutrient slowly. I believe the "pill taker" should be the "time releaser," not the pill (i.e., take vitamins at least twice a day, which already excludes some popular name brands.)

- Ignore multivitamins containing only 100 percent of the RDA. The RDA amounts just aren't enough to handle the many variations in people. The easiest way to select a preparation is to scan the label's ingredients for the one area (it's always there) that has the B vitamins followed by a number, (i.e., B1, B2, B6). If these numbers are all 25 mg—note that's mg not percentage of RDA— or higher, the supplement is probably okay.
- Vitamins should be taken with meals. There are exceptions, but multivitamins for beginners isn't one of them.
- No "multi" contains enough vitamin C. (I know of only one exception, so far.) The easiest way to add vitamin C is to get 1,000 mg capsules and take one twice a day at a minimum. (There are rare exceptions, so check with your health care provider.) Also bioflavonoids are desirable but not required.
- If a person can avoid refined sugar, refined flour, and fried foods, while eating slowly, chewing thoroughly, and taking the "starter vitamins," I usually hear about some improvement within one to three weeks. A "totally new" person? Maybe not, but usually there is some improvement.

What About the Dreaded Toxicity of Vitamins?

I used to tell a nonbelieving friend that I would be happy to compete with him, pill for pill in an interesting game. He could take good ol' regular aspirin while I would take the vitamin of his choice (C, B3, B6, the "feared" vitamin A, others, or even all of them together), and we would see who dropped first. Though meant primarily in jest, it's not a game I would recommend to someone taking aspirin.

On the other hand, I was actually told in medical school by a Ph.D. in pharmacology that 10,000 international units (IU) of vitamin A could kill an adult human. At the time my own mother had been taking 100,000 IU (yes, ten times that amount) daily for ten years to avoid a chronic skin problem. Prolonged lower doses would cause bumps on her arms and nose to reappear. Often, childhood acne will not respond to less than 50,000 IU daily.

Advertised fears of vitamins are rampant, both in medical schools and in communications to the public. Almost universally, such information is from persons who have neither seen a vitamin A toxicity, nor even used the nutrient as a supplement themselves, at least therapeutically. (*Note:* I would stay within a limit of 10,000 IU if it's a woman who's newly pregnant or trying to be.)

Anything Swallowed Should Be Respected

Nearly everyone has heard of the toxicity of vitamin A. About sixty cases, total, concerning this vitamin have been reported in the medical literature (yes, I looked). We're talking about side effects here—not deaths. On the other hand, few have heard about the approximately 600 deaths per year that have been reported from aspirin. Why is that? Could it have anything to do with high-power, wealthy, drug company interests?

Vitamins are about the safest substances you will ever swallow. They should be the natural form (except for vitamin C), as synthetic forms can be more troublesome. This is true of vitamin A, which needs to be natural fish-oil type. Vitamin E should say "d-alpha" instead of "dl-alpha" on the label; neither is toxic, but the body utilizes d-alpha better. Vitamin E has no known toxicity at any level. (Well, you could choke on the gelatin capsules, I guess.)

These agents are often even safer when taken together. For example, vitamin A taken with vitamins C and E has even less chance of causing any side effects (which are rare anyway). The B-vitamins should all be taken together before trying any individual B-vitamin alone, like B-6 for carpal tunnel syndrome for example. (They work better like that anyway.) Stay under 500 mg of B6, if taking it for a long time.

Vitamin D is said to cause a problem if you take over 400 IU (I'm becoming less and less convinced though) and really should not be in our milk (not that we should be drinking pasteurized, homogenized cow juice anyway). Natural vitamin D comes from skin exposure to the sun, and that's how it should be acquired (that's *exposed*, not deep fried).

Vitamin K can cause a problem if you don't know what you're doing, which is why few multivitamins have any and none has much, but it can be very helpful in the right cases.

There are no drugs I know of with the safety of nutritional supplements—the pain killers, anti-inflammatories, antacids, sleeping pills, cough and cold preparations, antiperspirants, you name it. If you fear vitamins more, you aren't informed about the drugs in your medicine cabinet.

So, I believe basically everyone should be taking some array of vitamins and minerals. I take them myself and will never voluntarily stop doing so. Am I wasting my money? Maybe. I don't know the perfect dose of each nutrient for my specific body (or yours), so I'm probably getting too much of some, not enough of others. I feel better on them, though. Lots better. Placebo effect? Am I better because I think I should be? Maybe. Do I have expensive urine? You bet, and I'm worth it. So are you.

CHAPTER 8

The Vitamins and Minerals

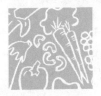

THIS CHAPTER IS made up of cameo appearances by each of the vitamins and minerals. That's all you need right now. At this stage of the game it's appropriate to know what's out there, but taking individual doses of these supplements is premature. If you experience what I think you'll experience, assuming you finish learning the basics, then you may wish to advance to more in-depth references that give detailed reasons to increase individual nutrients.

That's why we'll take a moment to glance at the general multivitamin preparations before the introductions of the individual players. The multivitamins are where all beginners to the optimum health arena should start, and it's where most advanced students remain for their baseline regimen. These are the basic team, as most nutrients interact together. A good "multi" saves a lot of shopping hassle (and a lot of swallowing!).

You may have noticed that vitamins in fairly high doses don't scare me. In fact, I don't think the beneficial effects even show up at all until you are well above the RDA (the Recommended Dietary Allowances of the U.S. Dept. of Agriculture and the National Academy of Science). However, there's another reason to stay above the RDA for the listed nutrients in a supplement. In multivitamins it's easier to get far more nutrient for the money. Compare labels with the common "drug store" brands. Often you'll be paying for the Madison Avenue hype!

Good multivitamins also give you a choice on the label of with or without iron. Unless you are known to be anemic, on a blood test (serum ferritin), avoid the iron: it can constipate, and it readily causes "free radicals," which are well-recognized biochemical bad guys in the body, responsible for aging, poor health and a myriad of other problems.

Get as many minerals as possible included in the multiple. These make the pills bigger, but they can save a lot of money and hassle, not to mention that minerals are as important as the vitamins, if not more so.

You'll hear this later, but speaking of pills, try to avoid them. I don't mean avoid the vitamins, I mean look for capsules instead of hard pills. Some do a horrible job of breaking down in the body. Why bother to buy them if you don't absorb them?

Again, a true beginner should not be starting with one or two individual vitamins; it's just too random a shot at whatever you're trying to improve, and it certainly is not your best shot, even if you want to "keep it simple" and just try one vitamin a friend told you about. Since nutrients interact with each other for improved effects, you're right back with a good multivitamin. Anyway, here's a very brief introduction to the basic players.

The Vitamins

B-Complex

These are the weird letter and number combinations (and some funky words), due to the fact that each interacts with each other: B1 (thiamine), B2 (riboflavin), B3 (niacin, niacinamide), B5 (pantothenic acid), B6 (pyridoxine, pyridoxal-5-phosphate), B12 (cyanocobalamin), biotin, folic acid and some lesser-known ones. Most of the time, beginners can remain in the middle of the aisle here until they know a bit more about navigating these shelves.

Single B-vitamins can cause relative deficiencies of other members of the B-family, so usually the multivitamin is a better start. There are exceptions, however—times when taking just one member of the B-family will be beneficial (see sidebar).

Vitamin A

This fat-soluble vitamin is good for skin, but synthetic forms should not be taken. Stay with "natural fish oil" forms. Beta carotene is a water-soluble precursor of vitamin A, with less fears of overstated toxicities, but not as useful for some complaints.

Vitamin C

We'll beat this one to death in Chapter 9 (though it won't die of scurvy!), so this is only a quick overview: vitamin C is amazingly versatile and as nontoxic as almost anything can be. Though its original claim to fame was for stopping scurvy, in higher doses it has been used for many other things, including accelerating wound healing, fighting viruses (including the common cold), controlling allergies, detoxifying the body, and strengthening the immune system. A versatile nutrient, but higher doses are needed for effects other than stopping scurvy, and many people often (and safely!) take daily doses measured in grams, instead of milligrams.

Remember the relationship between vitamin C and kidney stones because sooner or later a new sailor into health food waters will hear: "The vitamin can cause oxalate-type kidney stones." Jonathan Wright, M.D., the world's foremost expert on vitamin therapies, says, "in ten years, I've observed it once." And that was a high dose. See your health care practitioner before exceeding 3,000 mg per day. (You should see one anyway).

Vitamin D

The ideal way to get this nutrient is from exposure of the skin to sunlight (the natural way it is made in the body), so unless you

When It's Good to Take One Type of B-Vitamin

- Biotin is good for hair, without messing up any other nutrients, but they are very low-dose pills/capsules in the United States, so it takes a lot to get anywhere. (Other countries supply higher quantities in the pills with less filler, but they just are not available here.)
- Folic acid, or folate, should be taken in higher doses by women trying to get pregnant and in the first trimester to insure against neural tube defects of the spinal cord.
- Vitamin B1 can be taken by alcoholics and sugar junkies.
- Vitamin B2 may be needed if hair stays excessively oily.
- Vitamin B3 is good for high cholesterol without messing up the others, but only niacin helps—not niacinamide. A nontoxic event, called the "niacin flush," with tingling, redness, and itching (similar to a temporary sunburn) occurs with higher doses of niacin, lasting fifteen minutes or so. This effect normally disappears when taken consistently. Niacinamide has no "flush," and has been used with real success in cases of arthritis.
- Vitamin B6 can be increased, up to 100 extra mg, for carpal tunnel syndrome, bloating of the extremities, and/or premenstrual tension. Some people go higher, but you should read more on this fascinating nutrient first, such as *Vitamin B6: The Doctor's Report,* by John Ellis, M.D. (There have been reported problems with numbness and tingling in the extremities if this nutrient is used in very high doses compared to the other B-vitamins. Though the symptoms subside after discontinuation, it is worth knowing what you are doing.)
- Vitamin B12, which seems to help energy, may be taken anytime, in any dose, without messing up levels of the others.

are more experienced with vitamin supplements, stick with the amount supplied in a good multivitamin. Do your best to get thirty minutes a day of real sunlight, over as much of your body as possible, and without sunscreen. (You'll feel better, too.) It's measured in IU and 400 is the norm.

Vitamin E

This is a fat-soluble nutrient, and marvelous stuff, especially for those with cardiovascular problems. It is an older member of a group called the "antioxidants," which have been getting increased press lately as substances that help quench bad guys called "free radicals," in the fight to slow the aging process.

Check the label for whether there is a "d" or "dl" at the start of the chemical name (alpha-tocopherol, tocopheryl acetate, or something similar). The "dl" form is okay for topical use, but the "d" form is the better choice for oral intake, even though it is a bit more expensive. Now that "mixed tocopherols" are more readily available, I prefer this form.

As with vitamin D, vitamin E is also measured in IU and 200 to 400 IU is reasonable, though some people have taken much higher, and for many years. It is suggested that first timer users start with 100 IU; although rarely, the nutrient can have such a rejuvenating effect on the heart that blood pressure can briefly go up until the body gets used to it. After your body has adjusted, you can then consider increasing the dose. (Though admittedly very uncommon, it's always smart to play it safe, be monitored, and get informed.)

Vitamin E works even better with selenium, so you may find that micromineral included in some vitamin E supplements. This is a good way to get the supplement, as long as the price is only mildly increased.

Other Nutrients

As you might imagine, we haven't exhausted the list. We won't hit them all, but the popular ones should be mentioned. Further reading is recommended before spending too much money. Not that each alone wouldn't be helpful; it's just that you can spend a lot of money and not be sure which supplement did the most for you.

• Choline is a less-known member of the B-vitamin family. It is involved in nerve transmission and the utilization of fats. It is part of lecithin, a natural emulsifier and is rarely taken without equal amounts of inositol.

- Inositol is also a B-vitamin; therefore, it is water soluble and measured in milligrams. Inositol partners with choline in handling fats and cholesterol.
- PABA (para amino benzoic acid) is another water-soluble B-vitamin and is useful for healthy skin—especially those who have trouble tanning. This is ironic, since PABA was the original sun block in many sunscreens. A large number of people are absolutely convinced that high doses prevent gray hair.
- Vitamin K, a fat-soluble vitamin (measured in IU), is involved in blood clotting. It can be destroyed by aspirin and is seldom included in multivitamin preparations. Unless specifically called for, few people use this less-known nutrient, but it has become more popular recently in controlling the advance of cases of "spider veins." Some literature is also starting to appear concerning studies with this nutrient in controlling osteoporosis in postmenopausal women.
- Vitamin "P" is better known as bioflavonoids. The bioflavonoids are a water-soluble family of substances closely associated with vitamin C and should be taken with it. They are involved with the integrity of blood vessel walls, and subsequently with easy bleeding and bruising. Though part of a less-known group of substances, they seem to enhance the effect of the vitamin C. If you can get it without using a lot more cash, by all means do it.

The Minerals

In recent years it has become appreciated that the minerals play a more important therapeutic role than was previously thought—even rivaling vitamins. Though toxicities are rare, it's easier to cause imbalances with each other.

More important, unfortunately, is the fact that as a nation the U.S. is besieged with a soil-depletion problem. Poor (or no) crop rotation, synthetic (highly incomplete) fertilizers, years of pesticides, and other factors have combined to tax our soil. The orignal rich supply of minerals has been one of the greatest victims.

Minerals Are Available in Three Forms

- Elemental (Salts): These are the cheapest minerals. They are fine, except that they are poorly absorbed.

- Chelated: These are better absorbed, due to the fact that the mineral is in a specially bound form, or chelated (pronounced KEY-lay-ted), which is more bioavailable.

- Colloidal: These are the best in terms of absorption, but they are also the most expensive. Further, when higher doses are needed for specific reasons, it's difficult to find them in this form. Colloidal minerals are suspended in a liquid, some of which taste pretty bad, unless they are mixed with something else.

Normally, then, a beginner would rely on a good multimineral for day-to-day maintenance, or for someone trying to take fewer pills, a good multivitamin that contains minerals, though often the quantities of minerals are less than ideal in a multivitamin.

Minerals, as a general rule, require higher amounts in the body when compared to vitamins. Exceptions include the microminerals, or trace minerals, such as chromium, selenium, vanadium, molybdenum and boron, which are needed in the body only in microgram (mcg) amounts. As a group, they all work better when the vitamins are supplied. All these substances are basically available in three forms—elemental (salts), chelated, and colloidal (see table)—and it does seem to make a difference for absorption by the body depending on the form used.

Though a beginner should consider more of a multimineral first, this list is just a basic introduction to the minerals.

Calcium

This is the most prominent mineral and is well known for producing healthy bones and teeth, but it's involved in many systems, including the heart, skin, nerves, and many enzymes. It helps with

muscle cramping, nervousness, and tingling, besides bone structure. You shouldn't take calcium without a dose of magnesium at
least equal to half your calcium intake.

Magnesium

Talk about an incredible mineral. And incredibly nontoxic,
unless you have kidney failure (in which case you're a pretty sick
cookie). It's wonderful for nerves, muscle cramps and tension, and
it can be taken without calcium. High doses loosen the stools.

Phosphorous

Almost too available in the American diet, phosphorous is hard
to get too little of, but a deficiency could cause growth problems.

Potassium

If you want a good nutrient for heart rhythm, muscle contraction, nerves and skin, potassium's a winner. However, a health nut
seldom takes this mineral by itself.

Sodium

It's probably no news that sodium is so prevalent in our diet
as table salt that it is rarely added to many multimineral preparations, if any.

Sulfur

This is a major mineral for skin, hair, and nails, because it is
involved in the synthesis of collagen (the number one repair protein). It needs most of the B-complex at the same time to be really effective. Several forms of dermatitis often improve with this
mineral, especially when mixed with copper and zinc.

Zinc

This is the most popular mineral for skin and can be very effective. It is found in high doses in the prostate and is used effectively in conjunction with other natural substances to treat benign enlargement. It appears to play a role in upper respiratory infections and is used with vitamin A for short periods to shorten the duration of the infection. By itself, it is nontoxic in anything approaching reasonable doses, but high doses over long periods can cause relative deficiencies of copper.

Copper

Copper is involved in the immune system, hair, skin, red blood cell formation and the elastin of muscle fibers. It used to be all too easy to get high doses of this mineral when everyone had copper water pipes, but that has changed with the current use of PVC in residential water systems. It should be taken with adequate zinc, as they weaken each other's effects. This mineral can be involved in relieving iron deficiency anemia when iron supplements taken by themselves have not worked to alleviate the situation.

Iodine

As you know, this mineral works predominantly in the thyroid, but it also is involved in healthy hair, skin, teeth, and nails. Cold extremities, goiter, mental slowing, and very easy weight gain may benefit from this nutrient, though a thyroid test should also be done. Kelp supplements, often found in health food stores, are sold to provide this mineral.

Manganese

It is sometimes confused with magnesium, but it's a totally separate mineral. It is needed in brain, muscle, and nerve tissue. Also it is important in the reproductive process, including the mammary glands. Many enzymes require this mineral, and with vitamin B1, it may be very important for alcoholics, especially if muscle coordination is affected. Manganese should be used in lower doses than magnesium.

Iron

Though of course a vital mineral, iron may at times be less important than we are sometimes led to believe, especially in cases of fatigue. It's involved in the production of hemoglobin and in strengthening bone, nails, and teeth. However, as a supplement, it's a potent generator of free radicals, which are cell stressors, and which may accelerate the aging process. The mineral can also cause constipation and stomach discomfort. Many of the really up-to-date multivitamin/mineral companies now recognize this and offer their formulations both with and without iron. If you suspect anemia, see your health care practitioner, and be sure the workup includes a serum ferritin test.

Selenium

This is a trace mineral (meaning it is usually measured in much smaller quantities in the body) that helps work against damaging free radicals and their aging effects on cells. It helps in the production of antibodies and the elasticity of youthful skin. It works well with vitamin E to strengthen the heart.

Chromium

Another trace mineral, chromium is popular for good reason. In the battle against adult-onset diabetes, it helps with blood-sugar regulation and the utilization of glucose for energy. Measured in mcg (not mg), it can also help in cases of hypoglycemia (low blood sugar) and the depression that can accompany it. The most popular forms of this nutrient are chromium picolinate and GTF chromium (glucose tolerance factor).

Vanadium

Also called vanadyl sulfate, this trace mineral is finding a functional place in the battle to help control blood sugar. Together with chromium and sugar avoidance, it has allowed many type II diabetics (the adult-onset types) to lower their medication dosage levels, and some conscientious patients have been able to stop their drugs altogether. (Now kids, don't try this at home without proper supervision.)

Boron

A newer discovery, boron, has recently been shown to play an important role in the maintenance of bone integrity and, subsequently preventing osteoporosis. You can purchase it as an individual trace element.

Molybdenum

For those who can pronounce it, molybdenum is the last trace mineral on our list. It has been found to have a vital role for enzymes needed in the production of muscle energy. Also, blood levels for this mineral have been found to be deficient in persons having problems with multiple chemical sensitivities, as they seem to need higher levels of enzymes requiring this nutrient for normal function.

After such a long, yet basic introduction to the minerals, suffice it to say a beginner should stay with a good basic multimineral supplement until reading more about a particular health condition and its specific treatment.

CHAPTER 9

Vitamin C: The Super Supplement

"GREETINGS, FELLOW MUTANTS."

I received this bizarre salutation at a nutrition seminar many years ago. It piqued my interest, since remarks like that don't usually start my weekend. It turned out that the comment, though unique, was anything but inaccurate, and along with one other comment, it subsequently changed the way I looked at high-dose nutrient supplementation.

Background Information

We (those of us of the human race) really are genetic mutants, all of us. Each one of us has precisely the same abnormality within our biochemical make up: we cannot manufacture our own vitamin C, otherwise known as ascorbic acid or ascorbate. This places us in fairly limited company in the animal kingdom, since the guinea pig, the South American fruit-eating bat, and members of the ape family are the only other exceptions. (I think there's also a certain type of bird with the same problem.)

All other animals can make the nutrient from glucose, which is the common sugar in the bloodstream; this means that in them it's not even a vitamin. (By definition, vitamins are substances required by the body that cannot be produced by it.) When under stress—any stress—what is really remarkable is that the rest of the animal world automatically (and massively) increases its output of ascorbic acid in an amount relative to the degree of the stress. This can truly end up being a huge quantity, as you will see, when compared to what is in the human's diet.

Tying the amount of stress to the amount of vitamin C leads me to the other significant comment that affected me about this remarkable substance. It came from double Nobel prize winner Linus Pauling, Ph.D., who took 18,000 milligrams of ascorbic acid daily for decades until his death at ninety three. (I guess the vitamin C finally got him!) He said that if you take vitamin C, and you still have allergies, then you just simply aren't taking enough . . . period.

As I was on 3,000 mg per day at the time, and still having terrible allergies (for thirty years!), I was surprised. But, I decided to double the amount, which did not seem to help at all. As a last resort, I added another 3,000 mg to the regimen (9,000 mg/day!), and my allergies totally stopped that day, and stayed completely gone for over six years. (The symptoms returned after six years, from moving to a building where the inhalant stresses were too great for the vitamin C dose. They're again under control on lower doses, due to other changes.)

How can this be, if the Recommended Daily Allowance (RDA) of vitamin C is only 60 mg? (Or, rather, shouldn't I be dead, or peeing out huge kidney stones, or something?) What's going on here? What about those who take even bigger doses? If high doses are better, why don't we hear more about them?

Any fifth grader could tell you (prior to the destruction of our education system) that vitamin C is what prevents scurvy. However, the vitamin's role in optimizing the performance of our bodies is infinitely more involved than that, which helps explain why its production in ascorbate-producing animals is so vastly enhanced during stress.

Scurvy is, by definition, the end state of a vitamin C deficiency,

Two BIG Questions about Vitamin C Dosage

1. Why is there such a big difference in animals that, all religion aside, are so biochemically similar?

2. How can only one number (i.e., 60 mg) be picked for humans of vastly differing weights? The monkey's need was calculated by the kilogram, not by the ape. Plus, the 60 mg completely ignores someone with poor absorption, or other differences in biochemical make-up, who would have poor utilization of the nutrient.

and it's a horrible type of terminal event if left untreated. Collagen, the number one repair protein in the body, loses its ability to repair tissues, or even to continue to hold them together, including skin, tendons, the living part of bones, and all connective tissues, including the muscles, individual organs, and even the brain). The capillaries weaken, begin to bleed (everywhere), and the victim weakens, wastes away and finally dies. This state of affairs was the greatest killer of sailors for hundreds of years, and in 1577 a fully staffed Spanish galleon was found, at sea, with everyone on board dead of scurvy, right down to the last man.

The U.S. National Research Council has determined a level of vitamin C intake that avoids the overt symptoms of scurvy. That level is 60 mg, and has become the RDA. Except for gums that bleed easily, which 60 mg won't prevent, the other symptoms seem to be avoided; but that's all.

So, a glass of orange juice can prevent scurvy, and now you don't bleed to death. The real news of vitamin C, however, is far, far greater than that, with enough potential advantages to very likely give this substance the reputation of the most important nutrient of all time. This is where the bigger doses come in.

Is there any rationale for large amounts of ascorbic acid? Here's where things get cute. The very same National Research Council generates dietary recommendations for animals. When they got to the monkey, vitamin C was officially established at 55 mg for each kilogram (2.2 pounds) of body weight. When equated to the human (with an official allowance of 60 mg, remember), this works out to 2,500 mg per day for a 100-pound person, and 5,000 mg per day for a 200 pounder.

Animals that make their own vitamin C, like the rat or goat, when placed on an equivalent weight basis with the human, manufacture about 2,000 to 4,000 mg daily. Linus Pauling found that gorillas, who do not make it, eat about 4,500 mg per day, which corresponds to around 2,000 mg in humans. He also studied the foods that ancient man ate and found that our ancestors likely ate around 2,300 mg per day.

Why Worry If All We Ever Needed Was 60 mg?

Stress has been mentioned. The animal kingdom consistently shows that both physical and emotional types of stress have profound effects on vitamin C production—always increasing it. Ascorbic acid is a stimulant of the immune system, specifically utilized in the production and subsequent activity of interferon, a highly important (and very expensive) part of our immune defenses. Also, the nutrient is a strong antioxidant which, with vitamin E and others, offers strong protection to cell membranes in the body.

Vitamin C is also a detoxifier of drugs and chemicals that the body was not originally designed to handle. In high doses it helps convert these alien substances into a form that is more readily cleared by the kidneys. (Linus Pauling has done much of the research in this area.)

There is more. Since the vitamin is vital to the production of collagen (the number one repairer of protein in the body) all wounds, all maintenance, all new growth require vitamin C. Not only that, it's even an antihistamine in high doses, which is probably where some of its antiallergy effects originate.

Dr. Pauling has demonstrated over and over that there is an antiviral effect, including but not limited to the common cold. (Jonathan V. Wright, M.D., Frederick Klenner, M.D., Archibald Kalakerinos, M.D., Robert Cathcart, M.D., William C. Douglas,

M.D., and Robert Atkins, M.D., all published authors in the nutritional literature field, are examples of physicians who have clinically supported Pauling's work, and are highly recommended reading.) There are those who feel the Food and Drug Administration and the National Research Council are ignorant of the latest research on the subject of nutritional supplementation and what constitutes optimum doses, as opposed to mere survival doses. Others feel that since vitamins and other nutrients are not patentable, and consequently of low profit potential, drug companies may be having some influence on what research is being funded, and therefore what is being published. It is possible that the goal of finding the optimum dose of vitamin C in humans has suffered somewhat, if you subscribe to these theories.

If you are willing to buy the idea that the RDA of vitamin C is not enough, then new questions arise: Is it safe? Are there side effects? How much could or should a person take?

Safety

Vitamin C is one of the safest substances that a person could swallow. You can kill yourself drinking water, so I assume you could do it with vitamin C, but you'd have to work pretty hard. Some of the above-named physicians have repeatedly given upwards of 200 grams (that's 200,000 mg!) in less than a day depending upon the degree of ailment involved (severe viral or bacterial infections, snake bite, mononucleosis, etc.), with remarkable results. The really high doses are given intravenously (I.V.), but oral doses have been used up to 100,000 mg. People who were really sick showed no side effects and no toxicities.

One issue along the lines of safety has to do with the source of vitamin C. The very cheapest form of ascorbic acid (and it can be really cheap) is imported from China. There have been reports of small amounts of lead accompanying their product. At low levels of ingestion this may not be much of an issue, but those persons potentially interested in high-dose intake of vitamin C should seek the standard form of the substance, which is produced by Roche

Laboratories. Good health food stores normally can keep you straight, and there are also some good (and bad) mail-order catalogs. The really good ones often will tell you their source. (Good sources include, but are definitely not limited to, Solaray, Solgar, Kal, Bronson, Life Extension, Natrol, Alacer and Twinlab.)

Specific safety issues have been mentioned about ascorbic acid. One is that it might destroy vitamin B12. This was suggested in one study, which was performed by a known enemy of vitamin therapies and was found by Dr. Pauling to be flawed. He does not believe this to be an issue, and neither do I.

Another "concern" has been expressed that ascorbic acid enhances the intake of iron. What a problem! This just saves people from taking iron supplements, which cause toxic free radicals to form and should be avoided anyway in the majority of cases (even including many anemics).

There was a case, once, where intravenous vitamin C may have caused a problem in a patient who had a genetic defect in one of his enzyme systems, so if you are planning to have daily IVs of 80,000 mg (!!!) of ascorbic acid, get checked for glucose-6-phosphate dehydrogenase deficiency first!

One safety issue that high-dose-vitamin-C detractors like to mention is something called "rebound scurvy." The idea here is that your body could get used to high doses of C, and if you suddenly stopped taking it you might get symptoms of having too little. Actually there might be something to this, but understand what's happening: There are enzyme systems that gear up to handle enhanced quantities of C over time. These quantities are better measured in grams (where each gram is 1,000 mg). Once this pipeline is up and running, the body gets wonderfully used to having the higher amount, but can quickly empty the pipeline if more vitamin C is not forthcoming. Those taking high doses would not consider quitting anyway, usually, but if one decided to do so, lowering the dose by a gram a day helps prepare the body for the new dose.

Breast-feeding mothers pass vitamin C to their infants through the milk, so moms using high doses of this nutrient should avoid sudden switching from the breast to formula. As a matter of fact, switching to formula should be avoided period, but that's another story.

The only real caution concerning very high doses of vitamin C relates to the possible formation of calcium oxalate kidney stones. These very high doses concern bowel tolerance of doses of many grams per day (see side effects). Jonathan Wright, M.D., and Alan Gaby, M.D. (who have an excellent report called *The Ascorbic Arsenal*) mention that they have seen this occur only once in ten years, and they habitually treat with high doses. It is suggested, however, that persons interested in large doses of vitamin C have their urine screened to make sure that they do not have high oxalate excretion.

In addition, it is possible to supply "insurance" in the form of magnesium and vitamin B6, which not only are helpful in preventing the formation of stones, but also are recommended agents for a number of other reasons. (Dr. Wright and Dr. Gaby have a highly recommended newsletter called *Nutrition and Healing*, 800-851-7100; 978-287-2237.)

Side Effects

There are few side effects to vitamin C; and one of those side effects is even useful therapeutically. The most common is that of mild stomach distress from taking the ascorbic acid form, which is, after all, a mild acid. The easiest way around this is to take vitamin C as an ascorbate, which is a salt form and not acidic. (There are also buffered forms of ascorbic acid.) The ascorbates are sold as sodium ascorbate, calcium ascorbate, potassium ascorbate, magnesium ascorbate and polyascorbates (a mixture). Each is acceptable. The most popular form, though more expensive, is called vitamin C ester, or ester C. This is a much-touted trade name that seems to be very well tolerated in high doses. Whether it is worth the cost is up to the individual, but many people swear by it.

The real side effect of note, however, is called "bowel tolerance," and is worth understanding clearly because, if used correctly, it can be for a beneficial purpose. In fact, many physicians feel this "side effect" can be used as a marker for a therapeutic effect.

Small amounts of vitamin C are retained completely by the

body (though not stored for long). If you then gradually increase the dose, a point will be reached at which some of the nutrient is spilled into the urine. There is a misconception that any C taken beyond this point is wasted, causing so-called "expensive urine," a term commonly used by detractors of the high-dose theory of vitamin usage. The main thing to remember is that some vitamin C is spilled, but not all of it! Additional intake causes more to be spilled, but an additional amount is still being absorbed. For example, if you start spilling into the urine above, say, 200 mg, an intake of 300 mg might cause you to absorb 290 mg, while spilling 10 mg. Then, if you took 400 mg, you might absorb 360 mg, while spilling 40 mg. As the dose goes up, the percentage spilled also goes up, but you are still increasing the amount absorbed.

A final note on the good ol' expensive urine theory is that these spilled quantities of vitamin C are having a protective effect on the bladder. In fact, it's not at all uncommon for patients who have had years of problems with bladder infections to have them disappear, or nearly so, just by assuring that they are always bathing the bladder in "spilled" doses of ascorbic acid.

If you continue this progression, you will eventually reach a point where no additional vitamin is absorbed, and no more can be dumped by the kidneys. This is the bowel tolerance level, and it begins with the passing of gas, followed by painless diarrhea. Bowel tolerance of vitamin C is highly variable, depending upon the individual, but usually runs (pardon the pun) between 5 and 15 grams (5,000 to 15,000 mg).

This effect is not a sign of toxicity. It's a biological tolerance point and is used by many experienced nutritionists to find the optimum level of oral vitamin C intake, meaning they deliberately take a person to bowel tolerance, then drop back to the highest dose that does not cause symptoms. Some nutritionists even leave subjects at the diarrhea dose for a while to help detoxify the bowel of any residual buildup of undesirable chemicals or wastes. Observations made by doctors, such as Robert Cathcart, M.D. and Richard Worsham, M.D., include that of not seeing major improvements in disease states until a threshold dose has been reached and maintained. This type of dose involves specifically remaining close to the the individual's tolerance dose until symptoms clear, which can be rather sudden when using this therapeutic technique.

How Much Can/Should I Take?

Abnormal doses, obviously, should be given under the care and close scrutiny of a physician experienced in such use, as should any dose of anything taken outside of the norm. The debate concerning "the norm," however, includes the controversy of whether 2,000 to 4,000 mg constitutes the real normal amount that a person should be ingesting, since our ancestors apparently did exactly that.

My opinion is that nobody over the age of ten should take less than 1,000 mg two times per day, and others, like athletes under higher amounts of stress, should start at one gram three times per day. Normally, doses of 1 g (1,000 mg) twice a day up to 1 g three times a day, ensure a moderately high absorbed dose, while simultaneously and effectively bathing the bladder. (Bear in mind, these are my beliefs after years of personal research, but any conclusions you make concerning your own regimen must be made on your own. Read all the information you can get your hands on and make an informed decision.)

Whatever dose you choose, do not take it all at the same time, and do not take timed-release preparations. Vitamin C only remains in the system for a matter of hours, so you would want to spread the dose out over at least two times per day (the more the better). The only problem with timed-release supplements is that you are paying extra for a preparation deliberately designed not to release! Monitor your regimen yourself.

Often (along with the recommendation to buy timed-release), a customer will be told to take only doses from "natural" sources, like rose hips. Though I am usually in favor of the most natural sources, vitamin C is an exception. Most "natural" brands are predominantly synthetic, with some natural source mixed in for sales effect. If you can get rose hips at basically the same price, then give it a shot, but otherwise don't spend too much on the upgrade.

An exception, however, might be the bioflavonoids, which are compounds that accompany ascorbic acid in citrus fruit, residing in the soft, white area immediately beneath the skin. These agents, sometimes collectively called vitamin P, enhance the absorption of vitamin C and may even be required as part of the solution to some difficult cases of capillary fragility, where ascorbic acid alone was not enough.

Final Note

The subject of vitamin C fills volumes. You can never know too much about this incredible substance, and I strongly urge you to expand your knowledge base whenever possible. Do your own research, and do not let others dissuade you. So many times I have heard of "experts" telling interested parties that certain subjects are useless when they, in fact, have not even studied the matter themselves.

Read and study for yourself, then make up your own mind. Hopefully, this chapter may be the start of an experience with what I consider to be the most important vitamin of all. Of course, I think they're all important, but if I had to pick one, now you know what it is. If you decide to use it, I don't think you will be disappointed.

CHAPTER 10

Other Supplements

The Amino Acids

Bodybuilding

Anyone who knows a bodybuilder, or maybe even a weekend weight lifting enthusiast, has heard of amino acids, or "aminos": those almost magical substances for building muscle. It is not at all uncommon to see great big guys (great, *big* guys) walking out of health food stores literally carrying gallons of the stuff, in drums full of powder or jugs of premixed liquids, both combining many different types of amino acids.

Right off the bat, a beginner should realize that even bodybuilders may not fully understand the biochemistry involved here, though I admit most serious ones are well versed in nutrition. Combination amino acids are useful supplements, but they may not be for everyone.

Amino acids, the building blocks of protein, do allow for fairly fast weight gain, but gaining that weight as muscle calls for fairly heavy exercise. Calories from high protein sources, without high energy output are rapidly converted to fat, not muscle. The body can actually do this more easily than using ingested fat to make fat. What's more, there is a ceiling as to how much protein can be handled at one time.

For the skinny kid looking for a few pounds, read the labels, avoid as many calories from simple sugars as possible (these calories can convert even more quickly to fat) and stay under 100 grams per day, until you are well read (and maybe even then). I am not an expert on bodybuilding, but I have heard enough from those who are to know that there is a lot of controversy about optimum dose, even among the pros.

High protein powders are a mix of many amino acids. There are different types (simple, branched-chain, high-sulfur, etc.), all mixed and designed to build the most muscle the fastest. The jury on the ultimate mix is still out.

Therapeutic Uses

Individual amino acids have an entirely different purpose, and this is where therapeutic uses come into play, and where the non-bodybuilding public has generated an increased interest. What are they, and what do they do?

The amino acids' role as the building blocks of protein in the body cannot be ignored. The proteins in the body serve primarily two purposes: one is structural and the other is enzymatic. "Structural" speaks for itself, and all of the body's structures use proteins (even bone and teeth) during their formation. "Enzymatic" has to do with all of the chemical reactions in the body (which, as you might imagine, are a bunch). So these guys are pretty important. At the same time, unfortunately, absorbing adequate amounts can be difficult. This provides an even stronger motive for understanding what's going on and which of the substances one might need.

Eight amino acids are "essential," meaning the body cannot make them and must get them from food, while others (13 or more) are "nonessential" and can be manufactured from the others. There is some biochemical argument here, but we'll leave that to the big boys. Remember, nonessential doesn't mean you don't need it. Your body may do a poor job of converting the others, so you may need it badly.

It is possible to take enough of one amino acid to alter the balance with "partner" amino acids, though pretty high doses are required, and at times a change of balance may even be desirable. An example would be the body's ratio of lysine to arginine in cases of herpes simplex problems.

Individual amino acids, taken for specific effects, are a rare exception to the take-with-food rule. These are taken between meals, with juice or water, to avoid competing with other proteins for the limited number of receptor sites that are available for their absorption.

Types of Amino Acids

The following section is merely a brief introduction to the amino acids with known therapeutic value (there are others). However, now that you've had an introduction to the subject as a whole, you may even wish to skip to another chapter, especially if you already know that it may be a while before you'll be considering amino acid therapies. However, if you are, or plan to be, a bodybuilder with some potential interest in amino acid supplements, I recommend that you at least become lightly familiar with this list, to see that there is more to aminos than just a few pounds of muscle.

Our basic plan will not include amino acid supplements, either alone or as mixtures. I think it's important, however, to recognize

What Amino Acids Do for You

- Methionine (essential) is useful in increasing the growth and thickness of hair and nails due to its role in the production of keratin. It is called a "lipotropic agent," meaning it helps mobilize fat from the liver for burning. In this role it should be in combination with the B-vitamins choline and inositol.
- Lysine (essential) has been very helpful in the treatment of herpes, in doses up to 3,000 mg per day.

- Arginine (nonessential, but the body doesn't make enough) is required for herpes viral replication, and is suppressed by lysine. However, it is useful, with ornithine, in the production of growth hormone. (It is not to be used by children or by women who are pregnant.)

- Ornithine (nonessential) is used by body builders, with arginine, to stimulate growth hormone secretion. Take it at night on an empty stomach and it should have some effect.

- Phenylalanine (essential) has many uses, including appetite suppression, mood elevation, and relief of chronic pain. I have used it successfully many times in my practice.

- Tyrosine (nonessential) is used in conjunction with phenylalanine to cause an even stronger effect against depression.

- Glutamine (nonessential) is useful for mental alertness, memory retention, and the reduction of cravings for alcohol and sugar. In the form of glutamic acid this is a direct brain nutrient (along with glucose), but the glutamine form must be used, to first cross the barrier into the brain.

- Tryptophan (essential) is a sad chapter in the history of American nutritional nonfreedom. This marvelous nontoxic agent was used for years in the treatment of sleep disorders, hyperactivity, obsessive-compulsive syndromes, and even the tremors of Parkinson's disease. A single event of contamination, by a single company, caused the Food and Drug Administration to outlaw the supplement permanently, when (and this was proven) only the contaminant was responsible for some deaths.

- Threonine (essential) has been used to help the functions of digestion and assimilation.

- Leucine (essential) has been used for mental alertness, but is a less-known member of the amino acid family.

- Isoleucine (essential) is said to assist growth in infants and may play a role early in preventing some types of retardation.

- Valine (essential) can be involved in nervousness and poor muscle coordination if undersupplied. This nutrient is one of the less well known but is supplied by some companies.

- Histadine (possibly essential) is used in cases of allergy. Higher levels of this nutrient decrease levels of histamine in the body, so you might not need an antihistamine medication.
- Asparagine (nonessential) helps in energy production.
- Glycine (nonessential) is involved in the production of energy in the cells by enhancing the release of oxygen during aerobic respiration. A unique form of this supplement, di-methyl-glycine (DMG), was well researched in Russia for their high-level athlete programs with excellent results.
- Cystine (nonessential) is a powerful antioxidant that is excellent for hair. In fact, it is used in the sheep industry to increase wool production, along with other animal studies that showed high hair growth increases of up to 100 percent. (It's too bad these wonderful agents are not able to be patented, or perhaps a pharmaceutical company would already be spending large sums on a nontoxic potential solution to hair loss!)
- Cysteine (nonessential) is very closely related to cystine and is also both a stimulant to the immune system and a stimulant to hair growth. The amino acids both contain sulfur, which seems to have some bearing on their remarkable protective effects.
- Carnitine (nonessential) is not considered to be a true amino acid, but it's close enough and well worth some discussion. It comes from two other amino acids in the liver and is transported to the muscles, where it does a superb job of transporting fat into the cells for burning. Combined with exercise, carnitine is simply terrific stuff. For an athlete, it ranks up there close to DMG, but it's expensive and should be taken with choline, inositol, and methionine for the greatest benefit. For those who are not actively working out, the money might be better spent in other ways.
- GABA is a derivative of an amino acid, but it is also an important nutrient. It's used in the brain as a transmitter for nerve cells and is effective as a nontoxic calming agent. It's often combined with other nutrients to become a powerful antianxiety formula. (The actual name is gamma amino butyric acid, for anyone who cares.)

their place in nutrition, because it can be a very big one. It's just a bit technical to incorporate them into our starter kit, but more detailed information (both good and bad) is readily available. Body building literature is common concerning amino acids, but therapeutic information is tougher to find. Look for Carlson Wade's *Amino Acids Book* to start expanding your knowledge. However, if you want to know most of what is known on the planet, I suggest *The Healing Nutrients Within*, by Braverman and Pfeiffer.

Essential Fatty Acids

For those who have been tricked by the popular press, there are some very important fats out there, and very few of us get enough of them. This chapter shouldn't be a soapbox for discussing the problems with the low-fat fad, but it's important that the nutritional beginner hear at least one dissenting opinion amidst all the media hype. Certainly, many of us have overdone our intake of fatty foods. Unfortunately, the pendulum has very much swung the other way—and not by accident.

First, it's important to recognize the incredible attributes of certain fats (after all, they are called "essential"). The essential fatty acids, or EFAs, have been a much neglected area of nutritional therapies until the 1990s, when research on aging at the cellular level started showing the incredible importance of certain fats in both protecting cell membranes and facilitating a huge number of chemical reactions. Instead of showing up as just one thing, like the disease process of a vitamin deficiency, the EFAs seem to affect all sorts of areas, including skin (eczema, psoriasis), cardiovascular systems (coagulation, blood pressure), the immune system, fatigue, arthritis, menstrual problems, the liver, proper neural function in the brain, and more.

For example, one major area affected by EFAs is that of the prostaglandins, hormone-like substances that are involved in pain regulation, hormone functioning and the contraction of certain types of muscle. Almost daily, researchers find another reaction or function that appears related to the prostaglandins.

The list is long, and Mother Nature can make the point very clear: your body needs certain fats, and it can get very unhappy if it doesn't get them. Unfortunately, it's getting harder and harder to get them, as people shy away more and more from anything that mentions any grams of the "F" word. Not only that, the essential fats can be somewhat finicky.

The EFAs are liquid at room temperature, so if you find a solid form, leave it alone. They also go rancid (spoil) after a fairly short period of time, so look for dates on the label, and go with the latest.

There are two classes of EFAs. Both are needed for proper functioning of the cellular systems of the body, though one is easier to find in our diet than the other. As supplements, each will be readily available on the shelves of any self-respecting health store.

Omega-3 Fatty Acids

These are found in fish oils. The term *omega* is merely a convention cooked up to show the location of a certain type of bond (called a double bond) between atoms in a fatty molecule. In omega-3 the third carbon atom in the molecule chain is the location of this bond. For us, it doesn't make a bit of difference, as long as we can identify the name.

The normal oils on supermarket shelves have minimal amounts of these fatty acids, and it's hard to eat enough of the fish that have the greatest amounts of them. Also, the heating of oils during processing destroys the good stuff.

Brace yourself for more letters: the key ones are EPA and DHA. The letters alone are all you need to look for on the label, but for the local trivia buff, EPA stands for the chemical term eicosapentanoic acid, and DHA stands for docosahexaenoic acid. I use the letters myself.

Besides cold salt water fish sources (cod liver oil), the only good vegetable source is linseed oil, also known as flaxseed oil—visible on the shelf in both gel capsules and liquid. The linseed oil is easier to take as a liquid, as it has a sort of nutty flavor, as long as it has not turned to a rancid state when the taste clearly deteriorates. (This is the oil that has caused some controversy by being used in high doses in the anticancer diet of a German doctor named Joanna Budwig.)

Omega-6 Fatty Acids

As you now know, the omega-6 is nothing more than a different address for this fatty acid's double bond, attached to the sixth carbon in the molecule's chain. There are very few good sources of this oil, and by far the three best come from seeds of the primrose, borage and the black currant plants. (The only other good source is a woman's breast milk, but if you're like me, it's a bit hard to get.)

This oil is more expensive, due to the limited sources, but since many women are finding relief from the pain and cramping of their periods with high doses of it, suppliers are responding, making it more available at reasonable prices.

If you ever decide to try one of these oils, make sure that capsules contain 500 mg of GLA, the active component of the oil. Occasionally, a sneaky company will put 500 mg of the total oil with only a portion of that being the active stuff. Read the label. (See Chapter 21, "Navigating Those Health Food Aisles.")

It is important to keep in mind that all of these oils generate an increase in free radicals (the reactive molecules we want to guard against). Even so, the oils are highly beneficial, and we need them for optimum health in almost all cases, so this is not a reason to avoid them. The solution, then, is that anyone taking GLA, EPA, or DHA in any form should be taking additional amounts of vitamin E and selenium (or possibly some other antioxidant) as protection.

There are pamphlets on fish oils, primrose oil, GLA and the essential fatty acids, but full books are harder to find.

The Fat Debate

In 1990 I was in the clinic of another health practitioner (a homeopath) when he brought me an interesting article from one of his many "alternative" health care publications to which we both subscribed (but which we didn't both always read, I'm embarrassed to say). The article gave us a laugh, at the time.

Both of us had been preaching health for years. I particularly had given many speeches about a good diet and eating right. We both knew that fats were an important part of the diet, assuming you ate the right fats, and they even could depress the appetite, help control blood sugar and weight and treat a multitude of ailments.

I didn't give the article much thought until a week later, when one of my most trusted newsletters gave a lot of press to an ominous warning: The media, in conjunction with the new releases of expensive drugs to control cholesterol and triglycerides, was going to blitz the public with a major low-fat campaign.

That's when I knew it was for real.

Within two years everything was changed. Everyone was so "well informed" about cholesterol, triglycerides, fat grams and low-fat diets that anyone who said otherwise was crazy! Now I was not only a quack, but a crazy quack! It makes such sense, on the surface. Cholesterol is a fat; fat causes vascular disease; fat is bad; don't eat fat. Simple.

Too simple. And at best a half-truth. Has everyone forgotten what at one time everyone knew? If you eat sugar, and you don't use it all, the rest is immediately stored as fat! Guess what? If you eat protein, and you don't use it all, the rest is stored as fat! No one ever used to argue that. It's in every physiology text that's ever been printed. If you eat zero fat, absolutely zero grams, you will make and store fat. You will make and store more than if you ate some fat.

Many conscientious dieters know this. Very few people who really work on whatever diet they're doing this week think that the ultra, low-fat diet is the easiest way to lose weight. Very few. Most don't lose at all, and they feel worse in the process.

We've been had. There is only one way to make low-fat food taste good: add sugar. Sugar causes a much bigger release of insulin than fat or protein—much bigger. The insulin release enhances the body's formation of fat from those calories you just ate. It also stresses the pancreas, so that sooner or later the body may not do a normal job of making that insulin in the first place . . . not the best solution to the problem of storing less fat.

Oh, but it gets worse. Now people are so fanatical about eating a gram of fat, especially animal fat, that they'll do anything to avoid it. Margarine over butter? Margarine is plastic butter. It literally has artificial fats that damage the body. Butter is far superior.

Nobody ever talks about the quality of fats. Fats go rancid, stale, and at that point even "healthy" fats become bad for you. The unsaturated fats, the ones everyone has been told are so good, cause far more "free radicals," dangerous molecules that even the conventional medical profession is finally climbing on the band wagon about.

This mania increases the problem that is the focus of this chapter. Specifically, what is it about the essential fats that everybody desperately needs? Most people are not just cutting out steak, they are cutting out nuts, seeds, olives, olive oil, butter and more, not to mention being unwilling to eat any kind of oil on salads, flaxseed or otherwise, because it isn't fat free.

Cholesterol is used by the body to make hormones. Women especially need it, so much so that if they don't eat it their bodies will manufacture it. The problem is it's better to eat it, not to mention that small amounts of fat kill your appetite better than anything else. This is worst in teenage women, who are going through all sorts of hormonal changes and need the building blocks of those hormones. Now they won't touch 'em. (Like, no way man, I got a date!)

I am not in favor of eating lots of steak, well marbled and surrounded by an inch of fat; I'm against it for lots of reasons. I'm also against eating rancid fats, available at every restaurant that serves french fries . . . all of them. Once the fat is heated, it's bad, whether it's reused or not (and nearly all are reused). Hey, it costs money to throw out that pot of week-old fat in the fryer—let's use it just a bit longer. Add enough salt and nobody will know.

I'm in favor of recognizing that there is an important place in our diet for fats, and to some degree I include animal fats. Saturated fat is not quite as bad as we've been led to believe. Ignoring the low-fat mania is the better option—in my opinion, better than eating too much fat, which of course can and does happen. Chapter 20 lists the rules, which are easier to follow than counting every fat gram on every label and are better for you. There are things you need to look out for, no question. In this day and age, good health is hard to come by. There's just no need to make it harder.

The Herbs

In discussing herbs, let me assure you that we will not, even briefly, try to discuss them all here. There are just too many, and our beginner's guide would quickly become an encyclopedia. Besides, anyone using herbs, in my opinion, should acquire, and make a habit of using, one of the many good books that can be found on the subject.

It is important, however, to have a fair idea of just what's going on with respect to the more popular herbs available because they are not vitamins, and some of them should be handled with a considerable degree of respect. On the other hand, some of the improvements possible through using herbal remedies can be difficult to believe. This is definitely an area worthy of further study, and I strongly encourage it.

If you take some vitamins, and you feel better, there is a good chance that you are better. Concerning just a few of the more popular herbs, however, you need to be careful. The mere act of walking into a health store does not absolutely guarantee that everything in it is harmless. You can easily have the same problems, and worse, with over-the-counter medications from any drugstore, but people may not be as aware of potential problems in a place they may perceive as totally harmless. With those thoughts in mind, let's take a short look at a few of the herbs.

Ginseng

This is the number one herb of all time, with very little argument. (With my luck, I'll get one.) It has a several-thousand-year history of promoting energy, well-being (sexual and otherwise), clear thinking, and general health. It can be acquired in many forms, including extract (watch for alcohol), powder, tea, capsules, tablets, mixed in soft drinks and as the actual root, which is the only part used.

The Korean, or Chinese, type is supposedly stronger than the American, but you pay more. It is considered safe, but high doses for those who are pregnant or have hypertension should be avoided.

Ginkgo biloba

The leaves of this plant are used for improving blood flow to the brain, and several studies (done outside the U.S.) have shown the herb to help concentration, including helping the elderly and those born with Down's syndrome. This is due to a beneficial dilating effect on the blood vessels in the brain, which is more than just from a stimulant effect as with a drug like caffeine. (It is unfortunate that most of the good nutrition research is not done in this country, since the "deep-pocket" companies that purport to be into health are pharmaceutical firms, and they are not interested in substances that cannot be patented.)

Licorice

If you like the taste of this stuff, you are in luck because it is great for ulcer problems among many other things. High doses for prolonged periods of time can cause increased blood pressure, unless you get it in a form minus one of its active ingredients, glycyrrhizin.

Ginger

The root of this herb has been used since antiquity for nausea, including motion sickness and also morning sickness. More recently, however, it has been used with great success, in high doses, in the treatment of rheumatoid arthritis, as it apparently does quite a remarkable job of controlling inflammation. It is usually taken as capsules.

Garlic

Incredible stuff. The product of the cloves is used as capsules, powder, oil, pearls, and fresh for lowering blood pressure, as a multipurpose antibiotic, for digestive difficulties, and many other uses—though not as a breath freshener, to my knowledge. Put simply, it's incredible stuff.

Aloe Vera

Primarily used for burns and skin irritations, but it can also be ingested orally for a few beneficial effects. If this herb—fresh from squeezing the leaves—is promptly applied to a wound, it speeds the healing process.

Buchu

This is great as a nontoxic diuretic.

Uva Ursi

This is another safe diuretic. When mixed with Buchu, as it usually is, you have a great urinary tract cleansing agent.

Saw Palmetto

Also called *Serenoa repens,* the berry extract of this miracle plant is the source of the most popular drug for benign enlargement of the prostate (BPH), but using the natural form is totally nontoxic and completely free of side effects. (It must be the berry extract, and it requires at least 160 mg twice per day.)

Taheebo

If you like tea, try this one. Also called pau d'arco, this is good for people with chronic yeast problems. Mix the drink with some dark, raw honey and add some lemon juice.

Bilberry

This should be remembered by anyone with night vision problems. It is very helpful.

Gotu Kola

This is a great "brain food" by itself, and often it is used in combination with ginseng, as it seems to enhance ginseng's benefits. Gotu kola is not a stimulant but is commonly confused with one that is. (See kola nut.)

Kola Nut

This herb is a stimulant. It is caffeine, so compare the name with gotu kola. You will see this often in energy "pep up" products. It's cheating.

Ephedra

The active ingredient of this herb is available at any drugstore as Sudafed™. It is also called ma huang and is very common as an energizer, though there are efforts afoot to make it illegal. There have been deaths from this agent, some by idiots trying to lose weight too fast, others by bigger idiots looking for a "high." It is an adrenal gland stimulant and should be avoided. If you must use it, use a low dose, and let your adrenals rest by stopping it for two days out of each week.

Cascara Sagrada

This is an excellent laxative, but it should not be used habitually (as is true of any laxative). It should not be taken if the person is also taking the prescription medication digoxin, or digitalis, which is a heart drug. Cascara may potentiate or strengthen the effect of the medication.

Senna

The same goes for senna as for cascara sagrada.

Pennyroyal

As a tea, this herb is safe, but the oil can be very concentrated. In the latter form, which helps contractions during labor, it can induce abortion in an early pregnancy. I am told that the oil, however, makes a great bug repellent when applied to pet fur.

Stevia

Check this out as a noncalorie sweetener. It's expensive, but there is no aftertaste—and wow is it sweet! Besides that, the caloric intake is zero. The kicker is that the producers are literally forbidden to even tell you that it can be used as a sweetener. (Hmm . . . I wonder who'd care?)

Believe it or not, there are far more herbs than this meager list of the more popular therapeutic ones. Besides therapy, however, don't forget the more palatable realm of herbal teas. This can be a tea lover's dream, as their flavor is rarely bitter and very few contain theophylline, a stimulant similar to caffeine, which is present in regular tea. Most people scoff at the notion of herbal tea until they try them. Get a sampler pack of several flavors, and check 'em out. Not only that, some can be used therapeutically if you study them and know what you're doing. Not a bad way to take your medicine!

There are all sorts of books on herbs, in all sizes. For a good small one try *Herbally Yours,* by Penny C. Royal, at about 120 pages. In the mid size range of about 275 pages there's Earl Mindell's *Herb Bible.* (Remember that name. Dr. Mindell has been around, nutritionally, and you can't go wrong with anything he writes.) If you want the big Kahuna of paperbacks, head for *The Herb Book,* by John Lust. At 625 pages you should find answers to at least a few of your herb questions. It is also reasonably priced because it's a paperback. I'll remind you again in the Appendix (resources).

Antioxidants

This is a class of nonvitamin nutrients that has become popular as the concept of free radicals has come to light. Free radicals are molecules with highly reactive areas that interfere with many normal biological processes. Therefore, agents that intercept and "defuse" these molecules are desirable and are receiving more and more press. Some of the vitamins themselves are antioxidants (C, E), so it isn't a completely separate nomenclature, but here are samples of the more important nonvitamin types, though there are others.

Pycnogenol

Pycnogenol is a newer antioxidant, of a group called "proanthocyanidins" and is said to be much stronger than vitamins C or E. It is derived from the bark of a French pine tree, so as you might imagine, it is not cheap. It can be taken by itself and is nontoxic.

Grape Seed Extract

Grape seed extract is another version of the above, but less expensive, and possibly even stronger.

Coenzyme Q10

Coenzyme Q10 is one of the most remarkable antioxidants, as it is also involved in energy production in what's called the body's "electron transport system." It plays a pivotal role in all energy-generating systems. It's important enough that there are whole books written on the subject, one of the best of which is *The Miracle Nutrient: Coenzyme Q10* by Emil Bliznakov, M.D.

CHAPTER 11

Digestive Aids

THESE INCREDIBLY USEFUL substances have grown tremendous-
ly in popularity in recent years—and for good reason: they truly
are incredibly useful! Today, more and more symptoms in our daily
life are finding themselves linked to digestive problems, and assist-
ing the gastrointestinal (GI) tract in doing its job is becoming a
viable therapeutic regimen.

Enzymes

The body, of course, is supposed to make its own enzymes and
acids for proper digestion. The problem arises as the body ages
and it becomes less able to produce optimum amounts of each of
these enzymes and acids. If you ask for, or happen to find, the
enzyme area of the store, you will encounter all sorts of different
names: amylase, bromelain, lipase, ox bile, pancrease, pancreatin,
papain, papaya enzymes, pepsin, protease and probably more.
Don't panic.

The key for a beginner rests in only two questions: 1. Are the enzymes full spectrum? 2. Are the enzymes supplied with or without betaine hydrochloride?

Decision #1

"Full spectrum" digestive enzymes are those that provide the ability to help break down all types of foods—proteins, fats and carbohydrates. Actually, these are the minimum requirements. Truly full spectrum could also mean having an additional enzyme for breaking down cellulose, though this is not absolutely required. The human body considers cellulose a nondigestible fiber anyway and uses it as roughage, but the enzyme may be useful in helping to break down raw vegetable fibers for access to nutrients within.

So, if the label says "full spectrum," you're almost home free because that's what a digestion-conscious beginner would likely want. Then the only problem is whether the product is strong enough, which must be determined by comparing its label to others, and maybe by your own home trial.

Strengths are compared using the term "gastric digestive units," or "GDU." Look for these, and know what you're getting. Be cautious if they are missing.

If the words "full spectrum" do not appear on the label, then you have to learn just a few more tricks because the product still could be acceptable. These "tricks" are the words "amylolytic," "proteolytic," "lipolytic," and "cellulolytic." (Now you can read medicalese!) The suffix "lytic" merely means "able to disintegrate." "Proteo" stands for protein, and "cellulo" stands for cellulose. "Lipo" stands for fats, derived from the same root word as lipids, and you'll just have to remember that "amylo" stands for carbohydrate. So, a proteolytic enzyme disintegrates, or breaks down, protein, and so on.

If the offered product does not describe the above situation, then it's likely that you are looking at an individual enzyme, and not the full spectrum stuff.

Occasionally, an individual digestive enzyme will be used for a specific purpose, like papain for a breath freshener or bromelain as a nontoxic inflammation fighter in the treatment of arthritis. These are less common (though not ineffective).

Decision #2

Now, what is that other medicalese term, "betaine hydrochloride?" In short, betaine hydrochloride (or HCl) is a substitute for hydrochloric acid, the acid found in the stomach, though this source is usually plant based. It's not really an enzyme and can be purchased alone, but when used alone, it is not conducive to a comprehensive approach to digestive difficulties. Alone, it would normally be used only by those who know for sure that low stomach acid is the sole cause of their problem, or by those who, for whatever reason, do not tolerate enzyme preparations. Both situations are uncommon. Usually, benefit is noted within days—sometimes even less. Betaine hydrochloride is discussed here because it is so common to the enzyme products, and as such is an integral part of enzyme usage.

Digestive enzymes can be purchased both with, and without, betaine HCl. (So you're back to reading labels again.) If the full spectrum enzymes with it are tolerated well, that's normally how they are taken. I recommend taking digestive enzymes immediately after meals, so they only augment, not replace, the body's manufacture of its own enzymes.

One look at the popular press, and it is blatantly obvious that the common perception of our digestive difficulties has to do with too much acid. We are awash in a sea of antacids, for upset stomach, heartburn, indigestion, reflux, gas, bloating, the blahs, and blah, blah, blah.

In my practice, almost invariably I found the opposite to be the case, where acid/enzyme supplementation, along with instruction on how to eat properly, constantly paid impressive dividends. From the look of health food store shelves, someone else is finding something similar.

If someone has an ulcer, the conventional solution is even stronger: block all acid production with another battery of drugs (or give an antibiotic to kill bacteria that are only found in 30 percent of ulcer cases). Nutritionists are finding there are viable treatments that include two other digestive aids, where promoting "good guy" bacteria can be as effective as killing the "bad guys" (in conjunction with other modalities, especially including some herbal preparations).

A final note on enzymes. There are some nondigestive enzymes, the most prominent being SOD, otherwise known as superoxide dismutase. Its purpose is to break down the superoxide ion, which is highly reactive in the body, sort of a mega-free-radical, which has the power to do considerable damage at the cellular level and is implicated as a big factor in the process of aging.

Read about SOD before purchasing it, so you know what is going on because it's expensive, and there are other things a beginner should be doing first, though this is a good supplement.

Acidophilus

The full name of this item (as discussed in Chapter 6) is *Lactobacillus acidophilus*, but it is only one of many members of this group of substances. This is the popular name, however, that has pretty much stuck. Other names include *L. bifidus*, bifido bacteria, gut flora, gut microorganisms, intestinal microflora and probiotics.

All of these names represent living (hopefully) cultures of bacteria that are supposed to be thriving by the billions in the GI tract. The bad news is that they are finicky little guys and are easily disrupted. Antibiotics, hormones, high sugar intake, diarrhea and many illnesses can knock them for a loop, and they do not rebound easily. These products are as nontoxic as anything you can put in your mouth, and they are worth spending money on, but there are also a few things worth knowing before spending it:

• Potency is measured in "colony-forming units" (CFU), and these should number in the billions (with a "B") of units. You will find products listing millions, hundreds of millions, or sometimes nothing at all. Be careful to read those labels carefully.

- Chances are you will find most of these products in the cooler (though not in the freezer). Refrigerated is best, but just because you found them in the cooler doesn't mean they were shipped that way. (I don't have an answer for that one; I guess you just do your best, and take your chances.)
- "Active cultures" are the goal—just like you hope to find in active culture yogurt. (These are the "bugs" that will make milk yogurt when warmed and allowed to sit for several hours.)
- It is possible to find acidophilus on the regular shelves, labeled as "freeze dried." There is controversy over whether this is as good as the other types. If it works, it's obviously okay, but the only real way I know of is to use it as a culture medium for making yogurt and see if it works. Maybe you can get a yogurt-making friend to try it once.
- These cultures are also the bacteria that should inhabit a woman's vaginal tract, which is why many women get yeast infections after a course of antibiotics, which readily kills beneficial flora. (The stuff can even be introduced there!)

Different strains of similar bacteria may have different strengths. For example, one may survive stomach acid better, one may kill yeast better, one may crowd out bacteria better, etc., and some strains have multiple beneficial properties. One of the best researched types is DDS by UAS Laboratories, available in most good health food stores, but there are also other good ones.

There are reports of sensitivity to high doses of acidophilus. If a rash develops, you may have to cut back on the dose or discontinue it for a while. This has been seen even in nondairy forms.

FOS

This is the latest addition to the world of digestive aids and has been invaluable in the treatment of problems with yeast. The real name of the stuff is "fructooligosaccharides," so most people sort of stick with the name FOS.

The bad news is that this supplement is not cheap, though the price has been dropping as it becomes more mainstream. There is some good news, however, that is different from most supplements: FOS is sweet. It's a powder that is about half as sweet as sugar, but that's still pretty sweet. It dissolves readily, so it can be used in drinks and cooking. For those with sugar tolerance difficulties, this agent can be almost a deliverance, due to its main reason for being. The product cannot be burned as fuel, either by people or yeast, though it is readily assimilated by the desirable acidophilus bacteria. This offers a win-win situation, where not only do you get a sweet taste without calories, but also undesirable yeast are stressed simultaneously.

Still, we haven't even begun to appreciate the real advantage of FOS in diabetes and other sugar intolerance problems. To have a heat-stable sweetener that passes through the gut largely unchanged and without toxicities or side effects is an advance that should have a huge future.

There can be one small side effect in some people, which is that it can cause, at first, some bowel gas in persons who need the agent most. It's worthwhile, the first time, to start with a small dose (and maybe try it in private!). Then work your way up. The therapeutic dose is considered 1/2 to 1 teaspoon, two times per day.

Some suppliers now mix acidophilus with FOS. This is an excellent approach, in my opinion, though additional FOS may be required for full therapeutic effect.

That's the basics of Digestive Supplements 101. The rapid rise in popularity of nutritional therapies, and particularly in this area of GI (gastrointestinal, meaning digestive) problems, implies that it might be well worth dropping by the "health nut" bookshelves for a while to become familiar with these remarkably utilitarian and increasingly popular supplements. See the reference chapter for recommendations.

CHAPTER 12

Homeopathic Remedies

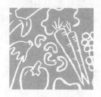

THE NUMBER OF POSSIBLE choices in homeopathy is even larger than that of the herbs, if you can believe it, and certainly every bit as fascinating. Nearly every self-respecting health food store has a section for these remedies, but due to the fact that the containers are so small, normally they absorb a much smaller display area in the store. Don't let that fool you.

Briefly, the therapy is built upon the theory of "like cures like," put forth by a physician named Samuel Hahnemann, early in the last century. He found that substances having the potential to cause a given symptom, in large amounts, could actually be used to cancel that same symptom, using incredibly tiny amounts. You must realize that we're talking about solutions so dilute that not even a single molecule of the original substance might remain, so there is no chance of chemical toxicity.

Homeopathy was very nearly destroyed in the U.S., due to the deliberate efforts of John D. Rockefeller and Andrew Carnegie, in the early 1900s. (It was never in jeopardy in the rest of the world.) The two billionaires cooked up a ploy to consolidate medical therapies into the far more profitable realm of patentable drug therapies, since they owned nearly all of what were, at the time, the fledgling drug companies. However, Rockefeller's personal medical practitioner, the entire time, was in fact a homeopath (*Health Freedom News* June 1993). Cute, huh?

The practice has obviously survived here, but solely due to the fact that the people who tried it got better, not because of any support from the medical establishment. As a therapy, it is one of the most heavily maligned, and only now is it gaining some degree of acceptance among those in the mainstream. In fact, now it's even available in many neighborhood drugstores.

Not that such a philosophy isn't easily maligned: imagine having your symptom relieved by a solution so weak it has zero molecules of the stuff that's supposed to be having the effect!

It's now known that one identifiable difference between a homeopathic remedy and plain water is its electromagnetic "signature," imprinted into the solution (Begley et al, 1988). For the curious, this "imprint" is produced by a process called "succussing," which is a special shaking technique.

Most homeopathic remedies are natural substances. Each is studied for its ability to cause a symptom or reaction when used full strength. Then it is diluted a number of times, and succussed with each dilution. These dilutions are usually denoted on the label by either an "X" or a "C," preceded by a number. The "X" stands for dilutions of 1:10, while the "C" represents dilutions of 1:100. The number preceding the letter tells you how many times the original substance went through the diluting process. So, a 6X solution, or "potency," means the original solution was diluted six times by a factor of ten, so it is now one millionth the actual strength of the original, with succussing having been done at each stage of dilution. The final solution is then applied to a tiny sugar pill or left as a liquid, to be taken orally (or held under the tongue until dissolved).

In this therapeutic technique, oddly enough, the more dilute the remedy, the stronger it is (higher potency), so a 6X remedy is more potent than a 3X, for example. The very high potencies (so dilute that the probability is slim that any molecules of the original substance remain) are considered strong enough that they should only be recommended and monitored by professional homeopaths.

There are over 1,000 homeopathic substances, with more being added over time. They are recognized as effective in a reference text called the *Homeopathic Pharmacopoeia of the United States,* secondary to either homeopathic research or long-term clinical use. Available reference materials allow you to research, to an amazing degree, the exact details of the specific symptoms a remedy may be good for. You don't just look up "headache," for example, except as a starter. The details can include severity, when it occurs, its quality, exactly where it occurs, whether it throbs, comes and goes, is made better or worse by other stimuli, and many more factors. Therefore, a remedy for headache may very well not do the job for your specific headache.

The types of symptoms can also be amazing. There are remedies known to do things like causing timidity and weepiness when music is being played. (This is quite a discipline!) However, many people who frequent health alternatives have found that over-the-counter homeopathic remedies for general symptoms can be effective, such as for colds, flu, headache, fatigue and many others. A fairly large market, in fact, has developed along just those lines, and is growing, so apparently enough people are getting satisfaction with the practice to continue it. It certainly is a safer effort than pumping down pharmaceutical drugs with known toxicities and side effects in doses easily capable of making those toxicities and side effects felt.

There are a few things that anyone interested in the study of homeopathy should know:

- The study is highly individualized. Good practitioners of the art study a long time, and a patient's history is very important to the resolution of many cases.
- For "simple" symptoms, such as colds, flu, and the aches and pains of everyday life, it is not uncommon for people to select their own remedies. You might consider staying with the weaker strengths, however, which means labels with 12X or lower.
- Remedies are strengthened or "potentized" by being diluted. Paradoxically, the more a remedy is diluted, the greater its strength. For example, a 24X remedy is considered stronger

than a 12X solution. The same remedy has been through 24 dilutions, while the 12X only half as many.

- Normally you treat one symptom at a time. The more traditional way even uses only one remedy at a time. Newer, and even computerized, methods do exist, and many therapists often use multiple remedies.
- For the more serious, or more long-term chronic illnesses, the use of homeopathy should be handled by an experienced practitioner. There's a lot to be said for going through the full history-taking process.
- There's no telling what the new labeling laws may bring, but for now the homeopathic labels are great. They tell you exactly what the remedy is for. Some mention specific organs like the thymus, the thyroid, or the adrenal gland. Most describe a symptom, like cough, heartburn, or headache. Others give a disease, like asthma or arthritis. You can even find habits, such as smoking. At the price, it's worth a try.
- There are mountains of excellent literature on the how tos. A good starter might be *Everybody's Guide To Homeopathic Medicines,* by Cummings and Ullman. Another good one is *Discovering Homeopathy* and *The Consumer's Guide to Homeopathy,* by Dana Ullman. (Mr. Ullman's been busy.) A good reference for treating at home is, believe it or not, *Homeopathic Medicine At Home,* by Panos and Heimlich. (The latter author is Jane Heimlich, wife of the inventor of the famous Heimlich Maneuver . . . just thought you might want to know.) Again, so you won't have to hunt all over, we'll repeat the book names, all together, in the Appendix.

A similar therapeutic effort using highly dilute substances is called the Bach Flower Remedies, which consists of dilute essences of specific plants that can be mixed and applied to specific emotional or mental symptoms. Examples include fearfulness, impatience, intolerance, shyness, sadness, guilt, compulsiveness and many more. In this practice, which has been around since the 1920s, liquid tinctures are sipped after matching remedies to a table of symptoms. The most popular, by far, is one called Rescue

Remedy, a mixture used for crisis situations that cause anxiety, such as receiving bad news, taking a final exam, etc., to relieve the associated apprehension.

As an aside, there has been considerable interest concerning the use of homeopathic agents and weight loss. This is obviously a popular topic today, with half the public concerned about it, which allows even homeopathy to get into the act (and legitimately so, in many cases). Recently, however, the marketing frenzy has included the use of transdermal homeopathic products, or "patches." These are homeopathic strengths (and are usually actual homeopathic remedies) placed by dropper on a small adhesive patch and applied to an area of the skin, usually a designated acupuncture point.

Though highly emotional results have been publicized (while nothing is heard of the failures), the American Association of Homeopathic Pharmacists has stated that the mode of delivery and the dosages involved have never been studied over the long term, and therefore are not considered official homeopathic remedies. I have no idea whether they work, as efficacy has never been studied, and though they would be considered far safer than pharmaceutical drugs, it is worth noting that long-term homeopathic-type agents may not be totally harmless.

If you try a homeopathic remedy, and it doesn't work, try not to run out and tell all your friends, "I tried it, and it doesn't work." Again, the practice is very much individualized, and people study long and hard to try to match the remedy, the symptom, and the subject. It often takes all three.

The topic is so large, in fact, that I hesitated to mention it at all. Hopefully, however, you will be tempted into health food stores as a result of the other things you've read, and you would then naturally stumble onto the field, so I thought I should mention it. Plus, the commercial interests are now getting into homeopathic remedies, so they're rapidly becoming almost unavoidable everywhere.

When they work, they really work well, so don't sell them short. Just remember that these are remedies, not to be taken daily, like vitamins. If you try them for something, like them, and plan on pursuing their use, find a knowledgeable practitioner (ask around) and work together with him or her. It will be worth the effort.

Modern Diet,
Modern Problems

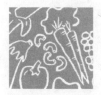

Tired of Being Tired?

IT'S AMAZING HOW a symptom that itself is absolutely painless can still be so completely devastating. If you have little or no idea what I'm talking about, then you are probably in excellent health and unaware of the extent of debilitation possible from being really tired—all the time.

We're not talking about needing a catnap here and there. We're talking really tired . . . trashed, crushed, wiped, zapped, gorked out—*tired*, all the time. It's incredibly common; and to me, that fact is really scary.

What's worse is that once you recognize your fatigue as abnormal (a truly pathological state instead of a normal need for some rest), there is a large list of possible causes. It's rarely just "iron deficiency anemia," no matter what your neighbor says, and sometimes no matter what even your doctor says. (Even if it's anemia, iron may not be the answer, or may only be a part of it.) However, see your doctor for an evaluation to rule out serious medical possibilities before relying on a purely nutritional approach.

So what do you do? Whatever the cause, you need a logical plan to track it down, because there really are several possibilities, and you should start with either the easiest or the most likely of them before considering the less likely ones.

The simplest is often the most likely, and that's the one that has been the primary focus of this book. Specifically, given the myriad of stresses prevalent in today's foods, environment and lifestyles, is it possible that you either do not eat or do not absorb enough nutrients to overcome your fatigue?

Assuming many of the "ifs" in Chapter 7 apply to you, the plan detailed in Chapter 20 should give you an excellent start on the problem. One of the facets that helps prove that this concept is valid is that, with the basic beginner's program, the same changes tend to improve a multitude of symptoms. This shows that the "whole" is a completely integrated group of parts that interact with each other when you do something right.

Of course there are specific problems and causes of problems that need individualized help for further progress. For example, a woman in her mid forties came in to my practice with not only fatigue but also difficulty concentrating, even when she felt fairly awake or was taking caffeine to assist her. The two are often associated, as you might guess, just from being tired; but this lady really couldn't concentrate, at all. She would go to work on her checkbook at one of the few times she felt up to it and find that she had been staring at one line for twenty minutes. She'd have trouble adding numbers that were long since committed to memory. (She came from the days when schools actually taught that stuff.)

For the record I start just about everybody out the same way, or close to it. That's because the basic rules are exactly that—basic. You get a team on the field, then you work on improving individual team members. The team allows you to at least play the game. As I say repeatedly, without the team, the greatest quarterback on the planet is useless.

Anyway, back to our fuzzy-brained, tired lady (she described her brain as feeling "thick"). She was willing to try almost anything, since she had tried most everything else and had been repeatedly told there was nothing wrong with her. In fact, what brought her in was the recommendation by the previous doctor that she needed psychiatric help (not at all uncommon in such cases). Not being willing to buy into that diagnosis, she decided to give me a try.

Her husband, however, seemed to prefer the crazy theory,

since he considered nutritional therapies to be about as crazy. Her diet was fine, his diet was fine, her blood work was normal, and everybody knew that vitamins don't work, so what's left?— the shrink. To fill this lady with both the basic routine and an additional pile of rules and pills to augment her therapy was just too antagonistic for her mate, who I believe would have dragged her out of there if I had added one more pill. So, we started with the basic routine. As you might predict from the fact that I brought her up in the first place, she got better. Her fatigue improved, as did her concentration, as did her fingernails and as did her allergies. The parts within the whole are interconnected.

However, the operative word was better, not well. I'm not sure she ever felt totally well, as in 100 percent of childhood, "life is wonderful," rose-colored glasses well. But, she was noticeably better, including in the opinion of her husband, and she wasn't done yet.

To get better still, it was necessary to then add the extras that were thought to be tailored to her specific situation. In this case an additional treatment regimen for systemic yeast, that her history indicated was a longtime ongoing problem, but which many doctors believe is a baloney diagnosis (or worse). And she got better, apparently a lot better. In fact, it was probably better that her therapy took place in two parts, so she (and her husband) could see and feel the difference and know what was responsible for what. Some patients aren't so patient. At this point I lost track of her, as many patients don't bother to keep coming back (and pay you) to tell you they feel okay. I'm just happy when I find out that a person stopped coming because they felt good enough not to need to, as opposed to because nothing helped. (There's always that moment of discomfort when an old patient stops me in the mall . . . what will they report?)

So, you start with the basics and see where you get, especially in the case of fatigue, which is such a wide open symptom with so many potential underlying causes.

Okay, you have a problem with fatigue. You've been on some semblance of the basic plan for maybe a month, and with a little luck, maybe you feel somewhat better; you don't feel great, but at least you can drag yourself out of bed with less than a fire alarm, and you can get through the day without dropping in the street.

What's Next?

1. A prime question in cases of chronic fatigue can seem to be a weird one: Do you sleep okay?

It's amazing how many people go to bed dead tired and then can't sleep well; in fact, some can't sleep at all. I don't usually worry whether it's a "chicken-or-the-egg" situation. These people are tired now and still can't sleep, so we need to do something. I have never found using drugs for sleep to be helpful; in the end, the patient awoke (or basically didn't) in such a "brain fog" that they might as well not have bothered. Plus there is no need for more drugs and more chemical stress when these people already have enough stress.

There is a lot you can do. Unfortunately, there used to be more you could do in the U.S. back when L-tryptophan was readily available. This is the amino acid mentioned in Chapter 10 that is amazing for both sleep and anxiety when taken in the right dose. Apparently it was too effective against the big expensive drugs because when a single batch got contaminated, the U.S. FDA outlawed all of the stuff. Only recently has it become available in the United States at all—now only by prescription.

With what's readily available, a great starter is magnesium. The 500 mg capsules, one or two at bedtime, can make a wonderful difference. During the day, those with anxiety can benefit from lesser doses.

In addition, there are some wonderful herbal teas with a therapeutic effect toward sleep. One that seems to work well is called Sleepy Time, but there are others. Just look around and find what best suits your needs.

A newer sleep aid, and one that has been getting a lot of press, is melatonin. I must say I have to jump on the band wagon here in terms of effect. Any doctor who says it doesn't work just hasn't tried it. Wonderful stuff. Having said that, let me add that I don't think it's for everyone. The smallest amount that works is the best dose, though it's certainly better than hypnotic drugs at any dose (3 to 6 mg is the usual dose), but if less does the job, use less. It should be reserved for adults over forty, in my opinion, as science that has no data concerning long-range effects. After forty, your hormone levels generally start to fall.

2. I deliberately didn't mention this one first: Could you have iron-deficiency anemia?

Don't assume this until you prove it with blood tests. It's the big catchall for fatigue, and everyone's quick to "pump iron," literally. Iron is difficult to absorb, causes constipation and dark stools, screws up tests for blood in the stool, and causes a marked increase in the generation of free radicals in the system, those bad guys of molecular stress. Be sure you need it first by getting a serum ferritin test. Your doctor should be happy to draw it for you. However, if it's low, he or she (and you) should be looking for reasons that you might be losing blood cells.

3. Here's the corny one: Could you benefit from a B12 shot?

Try one. If your doctor won't give one to you, change doctors. If it helps (or you think it does), get another one—or maybe even one per week. There is no reason not to. They're cheap, simple, and harmless; most people can easily be taught to give one to themselves. If it helps or you can't tolerate a shot, try the sublingual form available from the health food store. It can be almost as effective.

Even better is to have folic acid mixed with the B12. Your doctor probably should handle the mixing (or rather his nurse—most doctors mess it up). It can be painless and can be very helpful, even if blood levels say you don't need either one!

Ever heard anyone say these effects are a placebo, meaning you feel better because you think you're supposed to? Who cares? If you feel better (B12 is nontoxic), go for it. It's too inexpensive not to.

4. Could you have a thyroid problem?

Sure you could, so get tested. I also strongly believe that you can still have a thyroid problem when blood tests are normal. Try a book by Barnes called *Hypothyroidism: The Unsuspected Illness*, or one by Langer and Scheer called *Solved: The Riddle of Illness*, my favorite, for more information. (The riddle hasn't been solved, by the way.) If it sounds like you, take the idea to your doctor. There are also glandular extracts of thyroid available in the health food store. These have minimal active hormones and are controversial, though I have had good results with them, especially when mixed with kelp, which is high in iodine.

5. Could you have an adrenal problem?

There are different tests for weak adrenals, and I think they should be done more often because I think a lot of people have the problem. However, approach the situation with more than a shot-in-the-dark approach in this case. The latest youth formula to hit the market has been DHEA, the precursor hormone to a whole bank of other hormones. I love the stuff, and I still can't believe it has been permitted to be sold over the counter. However, I don't believe it should be used unless blood tests to monitor its levels are done, and it is not appropriate for those under forty looking for a fountain of youth pill.

Like the thyroid, there is a glandular extract of adrenal. The glandulars are slower to work, but they can be helpful, while being nontoxic at the same time. Still, read all labels and be aware of what you put in your body.

6. We mentioned this earlier: Could you have systemic yeast?

This is a huge topic, and we'll barely touch on it here. Though controversial, the idea is that years of antibiotics, birth control pills, cortisone, and other environmental stresses allow an overgrowth of ever-present common yeast in the body. When the patient's history suggests the patient be treated for it, sometimes the results are incredible. Responses vary in timing and degree, but most people with this problem feel changes of some sort fairly quickly. Bad cases do, however, often require prescription medication to kill yeast, like the generic names fluconazole or itraconazole.

The best book on the subject is *The Yeast Connection Handbook* by William Crook, M.D. See the Appendix for this and other book ideas if you think yeast may be part of your problem.

7. *Could your problem stem from allergies?*

Not only can you be allergic to anything, those allergies can do anything. It is not at all uncommon for any given allergy to make you tired; after all, it's a stress, and it's dragging you down, whether you're sneezing, have a runny nose, a headache, whatever.

Most people know that you can be allergic to foods. Except for rare, rapid onset stuff like rashes, shortness of breath, etc., most food allergies have long ago ceased to cause their acute symptoms. They only show chronic symptoms. That's because we often crave foods we are allergic to and can be sort of addicted to them, so we've been eating them for years and continue doing so. Often a symptom of food allergies can be fatigue.

Consider any food that you crave or that you eat every day a suspect. Give it up for one week . . . completely. (In the unfortunate case of dairy products, you must quit for twenty-one days.) If you end up feeling worse in the next two to four days, you are on track. That's right, and for want of a better word, call it withdrawal.

Usually, a symptom-causing food will be clear by day seven, and chronic symptoms may also be gone. Evaluate your energy at this point. You can then retry the food and see if it causes any acute symptoms now that it has been purged from the system. If you have found a food you are allergic to, eating it on a constant basis will cause return of the chronic symptoms. It's not uncommon, however, to find that infrequent ingestion of the food does not cause problems until you go over a given threshold amount or frequency.

Vitamin C can be a very potent antiallergy weapon. (See Chapter 9.) In higher doses it can do a marvelous job. As an example, I had a thirty-something male patient with the bothersome problem of chronic allergic rhinitis (runny nose). Though fatigue was also a problem, it was not considered associated at the time. After reading Dr. Linus Pauling's book on vitamin C and colds (this was early in my health nut career), I gave him a dose of 1,000 mg three times per day, which seemed like a lot back then. No effect noticed. As this was a man who wanted to be drug free I doubled the dose—a total of 6,000 mg per day. Still no effect. Dr. Pauling's admonishment, however, was basically that if you give C and allergies don't clear, you didn't give enough . . . period. So, my final effort (I was getting nervous by this time) was to increase the dose to 9,000 mg per day, in divided doses. The runny nose . . . chronic allergic rhinitis disappeared that day, along with a completely unexpected improvement in energy, and stayed controlled for six years, with no recurrences unless the dose dropped below some threshold-effect amount, which as that patient, I carefully avoid.

There are obviously other causes of fatigue, from too much partying to cancer. Some are just a bit easier to handle than others. The point is, you don't want to miss a solution that is not that complicated, may have many beneficial side effects, is inexpensive, and is totally nontoxic, with a not-too-unreasonable chance of at least helping. Even a total novice to the world of nutritional health can effectively give it a shot. The plan is in Chapter 20.

Decreasing or eliminating fatigue is an incredible signpost on the health-improvement highway. If you have been tired for years and your health program seems to have done nothing more than handle that, you are doing lots better. Consider it an email from Mother Nature.

CHAPTER 14

The High Road to the Right Load: Fat or Thin

WITH THE ZILLIONS of weight loss plans out there, I feel a bit intimidated making the following statement: Proper dietary habits will generally cause an overweight person to lose weight and an underweight person to gain weight—on the same diet.

How you eat and how you absorb are of course involved, but the fact remains that there is a good way and a bad way to eat, and the same positive habits make all people tend toward a norm. They may not overlap, or reach the same weight, but skinny and over-weight will head in the right direction. (The details of proper diet, how to eat, and how to absorb may be found in Chapter 20.)

Most people, though, are not at that "ideal weight," be it too high or too low, and might like a few hints that are more specific for starting the trend in the right direction.

First, however, one reminder: Don't get too obsessed with the ideal weight concept. Never forget that each of us is different. Some of you will never have a pencil figure, and some others will always have to work at filling out a normal size. First find out that you do have the ability to head toward your normal range, then let your fashion sense help you achieve some of the final polish that your genetic makeup may not have provided.

Gaining Weight

For the underweight, no matter what they eat, it just doesn't seem to stick. Though for many it seems like sort of a nonproblem, individuals trying to beef up a bit find it just as frustrating as trying to lose.

I have found that the most important factor inhibiting weight gain seems to be malabsorption and maldigestion. This is similar to those who are overweight, where foods may be absorbed enough to be stored, but not enough to be burned properly. For the underweight, they may not even get that far; it's neither stored nor burned, but just passes on through. What little they do get is rapidly burned by a fast metabolism, starved for fuel.

Everyone is different. A really jacked up metabolism can burn anything, no matter how it's absorbed. That's why thyroid hormone causes people to lose weight. It works fine, but the price to pay in side effects (osteoporosis, heart stress, others) isn't worth going outside the normal range. There are many, however, who are very slightly (or subclinically) under the normal range. They can benefit beautifully from low doses of natural thyroid by prescription. (To see if you are a candidate, try *Solved: The Riddle of Illness*, by Langer & Scheer.)

For the poor absorber, however, an excellent avenue that may be pursued is that of digestive enzymes (see Chapter 11). Taken after meals they do not inhibit the body's normal production of these substances and can really enhance the digestion, especially if the person eats slowly and chews thoroughly. That way the part of digestion that is supposed to start in the mouth has a chance to be properly performed.

Some people have systems that are so "hyper" that their transit time through the intestinal tract is faster than it should be. For some it's so fast they are even plagued by diarrhea, having what may be called an irritable bowel.

Even this can be slowed somewhat, without the aid of drugs (which do exist for the purpose). *L. acidophilus* (Chapter 11) in capsules, powder, or liquid form help calm the irritability.

Whether from irritable bowel syndrome or from surgical shortening of the gut for whatever reason (Crohn's disease, lymphomas, colon cancer, etc.), some of the thinnest people may have what's called "the dumping syndrome," where diarrhea is very common. Apple pectin works well here. It's available in powder form at health food stores and grocery stores that sell items for home canning. A teaspoon before meals can slow the action down without interfering with other processes.

Sometimes food allergies keep the gastrointestinal (GI) tract in such a turmoil that the body can't do its job correctly. Any foods that are craved, and any others that are eaten nearly every day should be tested by discontinuing them for seven days. If you feel worse from days two to four, you are on the right track and should continue, usually. That is most likely withdrawal, and you should feel better before the end of the seven days.

Unfortunately, often this problem is caused by dairy products, especially milk and cheese—less so with butter, and even less with yogurt. Any of them may be involved. This is not the same as lactose intolerance, though that does happen and can be handled with popular lactase enzyme tablets. The true sensitivity will not respond to these tablets. What makes the dairy sensitivity so unfortunate, besides the fact that dairy is everywhere, is that it must be tested for twenty-one days instead of just seven.

There are also those who eat huge quantities of calories as carbohydrates and gain absolutely nothing at all. These skinny types have a problem with their blood sugar. When given less sugar and less white flour, both very high calorie, and then given more protein, some fat, and naturally high-fiber carbohydrates (unrefined), these people start to gain. When this does happen, these people do even better with chromium picolinate added as a supplement. I've observed these people gain weight even though there were the same or fewer calories overall. Go figure.

Losing Weight

The problem with weight loss is clearly much larger (sorry). It's not getting any less, either; it's increasing. For the first time in the history of the United States, the overweight now number over 50 percent of the population as a whole. In the Associated Press release we mentioned in chapter 1, the writer said it best: "Flab is now the norm". For the first time, overweight Americans out-number normal-size ones, according to U.S. government statistics" (*The Arizona Republic* Oct. 16,1996).

Moreover, in 1995 the *Journal of the American Dietetic Association* (#95 417–420) reported in a chart that from 1960 to 1990 the percent of dietary calories from fat decreased from over 40 percent to under 35 percent. Over the same period, the percent of overweight people increased from under 25 percent to over 33 percent. We all know the media blitz about low fat. There is certainly less eaten in 2001 than in 1996, yet now our overweight population has burgeoned from 33 percent to over 50 percent.

What is going on here? It has always been obvious to me that fat is not the answer, and I'm no genius. Anyone who remembered any sophomore physiology course knows that both protein and carbohydrate convert to fat—and readily so. The refined carbohydrates do it the fastest because they cause the heaviest release of insulin, which builds fat.

Robert Atkins, M.D., "discovered" it over twenty-five years ago and proved it with thousands of people losing major amounts of weight on his high-protein diet (not just water weight, and without killing 'em, like his detractors love to claim). His *Dr. Atkins' Diet Revolution* was exactly that.

Now, go look at almost any low-fat food. They're even advertising candy bars as low fat! Well, it's true, why not? Check out the grams of carbohydrates on the labels to find the reason that low-fat diets don't work. Low-fat foods taste bad (plus they don't depress the appetite for any appreciable time), so they are loaded up with sugar. Your insulin levels go up, the sugar is shoved out of the bloodstream, mostly into fat cells, and away you go. Your blood sugar then plummets too rapidly from all the insulin, and (guess what?) you get hungry again. Then you buy more low-fat food. Cute. Stay with the foods man was originally designed to eat.

The one big subset of products not discussed in Section 2 is weight-loss agents, mainly because many are not necessarily nutri-

Navigating Weight-Loss Aisles

The weight-loss products are hard to miss in a health food store; they are often up front, surrounded by lots of ink. This is as expected in the U.S. and other "civilized diet" nations, given the current preoccupation with weight by both sexes, plus the fact that we are a fatter population than ever before. There's also another reason: Some of these products work. That's the good news. Just from looking around it's obvious that some of them don't. Of the effective ones it's important to recognize that there is a bit more to the story, and that many of these products deserves some respect. Some contain agents that, even though natural, may be more drug-like than nutrient-like in their effects.

Here are some guidelines for smooth sailing through the weight-loss products.

1. Homeopathic weight loss products are safe to try anytime, as long as there's nothing else in them. Usually this is not an issue, as they work better alone and are normally formulated that way. (See Chapter 12.)

2. Some products use high-fiber ingredients, usually taken before meals, to fill the dieter up and lessen the subsequent caloric intake of the ensuing meal. (Since fiber is not absorbed, it therefore has no caloric value.) These are okay, if you look out for other ingredients and take them with plenty of water. Also, don't go overboard . . . tons of fiber not only can act like an anchor but also can interfere with nutrient absorption. Once you lose the undesired ballast, let go of the anchor and maintain your smooth sailing with a food-only maintenance diet. If (for some totally unknown reason!) some of the weight starts to return, then you can reinstitute a short-term system early.

3. Be careful with the meal-replacement drinks or milk shakes. They can be okay in a pinch (like you're about to be lured onto the rocks by a siren holding jelly doughnuts), but they are expensive, and must be scrutinized closely for sugar, including corn syrup, sucrose, fructose, glucose, and dextrose.

These work by depressing the appetite, but rarely do they hold until the next meal. Normally, the worse they taste, the better they are for you, and vice versa, due to less sweeteners.

4. By far the most popular weight loss modality is thermogenics, usually, but not always, using herbs (see Chapter 12). These can work very well, and they have some solid scientific evidence to back them up. However, they need to be well understood, because what makes them work is not a vitamin-like mechanism.

5. All thermogenic products stimulate the adrenal gland and raising the body's metabolic set point, often by using different combinations of herbs like guarana, ma huang (ephedra), white willow, and possibly some form of theophylline.

6. To be effective, whatever the plant names, the formulation must contain some form of caffeine, ephedrine, and/or theophylline, plus usually a salicylate (aspirin), which slows the breakdown of the other three agents. Though potentially effective, I hope you are getting the idea that these products not only are not mere vitamins but also are not entirely harmless.

7. Some companies will add nutrients like chromium, some vitamins, and/or more herbs, but to be "thermogenic" the basic formulations will be similar.

8. Remember that the adrenals are being stimulated while on these products. Therefore, you should take a break to allow rest for the adrenal glands. Five days on and two days off is an easy way to remember. Then, once the weight is down, lower or preferably discontinue the product.

tional. The interest in them is so prominent, however, that we discuss them in this chapter (in the accompanying sidebar), instead of in Chapter 21. It will be sort of an early cruise through the health food aisles, introducing you to their weight-loss products.

There is one type of weight-loss product you won't find in the health food aisles, and that's prescription drugs, along with the the lower dose, but similar chemistry, over-the-counter ones. Be careful. These agents cause tolerance and rebound, meaning you must keep taking more for the same effect until one day the effect stops completely. That's when the the often harmful rebound begins. Witness the now-defunct phen-fen craze. Enough said.

A Quick Weight-Loss Plan

As an attempt to keep as many overweight people off as many drugs as possible, I offer an "enhancement routine" in addition to the basic plan presented in Chapter 20 in terms of losing weight. Most of it I did not think of myself (like everything else), but I have used it with considerable success, so I'll describe the technique, plus my little twist on it.

You may have heard of it. It's called the "Cabbage Soup Diet," and you only do it for one week at a time. I've seen different versions of it, but I believe that the original credit goes to Sacred Heart Memorial Hospital (I can't even find the city), which used it for overweight heart patients before surgery.

Actually, one twist I've discovered is that, when it works, it works nearly as well with French onion soup, too (go light on the salt, and of course the cheese and crouton are out). However, it is printed below as I received it with the exceptions of one omission and added metric conversions.

I don't understand the diet. When it works, meaning for those who can tolerate the week without cheating, the thing is amazing. You can eat all you want, so you should never be hungry—and the weight usually just falls off. Most people can't even get all the meat down before getting full.

This is all without exercise (though I do recommend regular exercise), and the weight goes away. I tried checking the caloric intake and gave up. Those who lose weight must just eat more calories normally than I ever realized. The idea is to do it for a week, then use the standard "good-eating" rules for several weeks. Then, if you wish, you can repeat it. That way it's safe—and not boring. Heck, you can almost hold your breath for one little week!

No one diet works for everyone. There is too much biochemical individuality out there for that to ever happen. And some people simply cannot handle the routine, even for a week, be it food sensitivity, inability to get or remain satiated, or whatever. All is not necessarily lost for most of these people.

My little twist, then, is this: Those who find the diet intolerable tend to be those who would do very well on foods of the Atkins type, high-protein diet (I'm not one of them, but I'm skinny so I guess it doesn't matter.). Foods in this plan include eggs, meats, fish, fowl, butter, hard cheeses, mayonnaise, nuts, seeds, leafy salad-type vegetables, and some heavy cream. For continued use of such a plan, plus recipes, I refer you to *The New Atkins Diet Revolution,* by Robert Atkins, M.D. Either way, most everyone now has a one-week plan they can use to start the weight-loss ball really rolling.

I don't leave anyone on either diet. You do one of them for one week, and switch to the basic rules in Chapter 20. I don't believe we were meant to be totally vegetarian, nor do I believe we were meant to have an extremely high animal intake (with a few notable exceptions, like some epileptics and some insulin-resistant diabetics). But that's a personal bias. How you follow the basic routine is really up to you.Good luck!

The Cabbage Soup Diet

You have been so good. You've been working out, watching the fats, eating lots of good food and no junk. Yet those last few pounds just won't come off. What do you do? Try the "Cabbage Soup Diet" and see what happens. Follow the instructions to the letter.

Cabbage Soup Recipe

6 large green onions	2 green peppers
1 large head cabbage	1 bunch celery
1 or 2 cans tomatoes	1 pkg. Lipton soup mix

Season with salt, pepper, parsley, bouillon or hot sauce.

Cut vegetables in small pieces. In large pot, add vegetables and soup mix, cover with water. Boil rapidly for ten minutes. Cut heat and simmer until vegetables are tender.

This soup can be eaten anytime you are hungry. Eat as much as you want, whenever you want. The soup will add no calories. The more you eat the more you will lose. Fill a thermos in the morning if you will be away during the day. Remember though, that if this soupd is eaten alone for indefinite periods, you will suffer malnutrition.

Day One (Monday)

All fruits except bananas. Cantaloupe and watermelon are lower in calories than most fruits. Eat only the soup and fruits. For drinks—unsweetened tea, cranberry juice or water.

Day Two (Tuesday)

All vegetables. Eat until you are completely stuffed with all fresh, raw or canned vegetables. Try to eat green leafy veggies and stay away from dry beans, peas, and corn. Also eat the soup. At dinner time, reward yourself with a big baked potato and butter. Do not eat any fruits.

Day Three (Wednesday)

Eat all the soup, fruits and vegetables you want. Do not have a baked potato! If you have eaten for three days, as above, and have not cheated, you will find you have lost 5 to 7 pounds (2 to 3 kg).

Day Four (Thursday)

Bananas and skim milk. Eat as many as three bananas and drink as many glasses of water as you can on this day along with the soup. Bananas are high in calories and carbohydrates and so is the milk, but on this particular day your body will need potassium and carbohydrates, protein and calcium, to lessen your craving for sweets.

Day Five (Friday)

Beef and tomatoes. You may have 10 to 20 ounces (285 to 570 g) of beef and a can of tomatoes or as many as six fresh tomatoes on this day. Try to drink six to eight glasses of water to wash away the uric acid in your body. Eat the soup at at least once today.

Day Six (Saturday)

Beef and veggies. Eat to your heart's content of the beef and veggies today. You can have two or three steaks if you like with leafy green vegetables, but no baked potato. Be sure and eat the soup once today.

Day Seven (Sunday)

Brown rice, unsweetened fruit juice and vegetables. Stuff yourself. Eat the soup at least once.

After only seven days of this diet, you will begin to feel lighter by at least 10 and possibly 17 pounds (4.5 to 7.7 kg), having an abundance of energy. Continue this plan as long as you wish and feel the difference.

This diet is fast, fat burning and the secret is that you will burn more calories than you take in. It will flush your system of impurities and give you a feeling of well-being. This diet does not lend itself to drinking any alcoholic beverages at any time because of the removal of fat build up in your system. Go off the diet for at least twenty-four hours before any intake of alcohol.

Because everyone's digestive system is different, this diet will affect everyone differently. After day three, you will have more energy than when you began if you did not cheat. If after being on the diet for several days you find your bowel movements have changed, eat a cup of bran or fiber. Although you can have black coffee with this diet, you may find you don't need caffeine after the third day.

Definite "No-No's"

Avoid bread, alcohol, carbonated drinks, including diet drinks. Stick with water, unsweetened tea, black coffee, unsweetened fruit juices, cranberry juice and skim milk (if you really have to have cow's milk).

The cabbage soup can be eaten anytime you feel hungry. Eat as much as you wish. Remember, the more you eat the more you lose. No fried foods or bread. You can eat broiled or baked chicken instead of meat (absolutely no skin on the chicken). If you prefer, you can substitute broiled fish for beef on only one of the beef days. You need high protein from the beef the other day.

Prescribed medication will not hurt you on this diet.

CHAPTER 15

Heart Smart

AT THE TIME of the Civil War, medical texts of the era did not, I'm told, even mention cardiovascular disease, with the first description of a heart attack showing up in the Journal of the American Medical Association in 1908.

Today, heart disease is the number one (that's *#1*) killer in the U.S. today, and not by a nose. Combine cancer deaths (the number-two killer), all accidents and homicides, and it's still number one (U.S. Census Bureau 2000).

Not to beat a cliché to death, but what's wrong with this picture? A nonexistent disease a century ago is now so prominent that even a beginner's guide like this book would be remiss not to mention it. (*Note:* That may also be the case with cancer, but we'll just have to be remiss there . . . nutrition and cancer are definitely linked, but once your immune system is depressed enough to get cancer it ceases to be a beginner's topic. Cancer, at that point, mandates an aggressive, controlled approach under the care of a dedicated professional. For ideas along alternative lines, I'd recommend the book, *Alternative Medicine: The Definitive Guide,* by the Burton Goldberg Group. Many different modalities are discussed, and clinics are listed. Another excellent and comprehensive introduction to alternative treatments for cancer is *The Cancer Solution,* by Robert Willner, M.D., Ph.D.)

So in the United States, heart disease raced from the back of the pack to become absolute front-runner in less than a century. But the citizens are told that their diet is the finest on Earth, with the single exception of eating too much animal fat.

However, decades of research by two amazing medical professionals leave us with considerable food for thought (if not for actual consumption) concerning the dietary fat issue. Weston A. Price, D.D.S., and Francis M. Pottenger, M.D., established that animal fat is just the type our ancestors ate fairly large amounts of for millennia without heart disease! Treasure troves of their work can be found at the Weston A. Price Foundation (www.westonaprice.org, 202-333-HEAL, fax: 202-333-0002), and at the Price-Pottenger Nutrition Foundation (www.price-pottenger.org, 800-FOODS-4-U, 619-462-7600).

There has to be more to it. Do we just work too hard (yeah, it's stress, like our ancestors never had it), and not get enough exercise?

Maybe. There are other accepted major risk factors: high blood pressure (but from where?); cigarette smoking (but that's been around longer than 100 years); male sex (but is that new?); family history of heart disease (but where did they get it?); obesity (with the finest diet on Earth?); and diabetes (now there's something, but why is it higher now than ever before?)

Given that all these are contributing factors, to say that the "fuel" in our tank is the best, with no need for dietary supplements, flirts with the absurd.

We cannot possibly cover a comprehensive nutritional approach to heart disease in a few pages, as there are heated dietary arguments and lots of supplement possibilities. Even a cursory look at health-nut sources reveals a large list of supplements for cardiovascular health, as the list in the table illustrates. This list is not comprehensive; there are a lot more. Don't panic, we're going to select from this list some of the most prominent nutrients as a nutritional heart insurance policy.

Heart disease is built around the general occurrence of fatty material becoming deposited in blood vessel walls. If such deposits

Supplements for Cardiovascular Health

Fat-Soluble Vitamins
Vitamins A, D, E

Amino Acid Type Compounds
L-Carnitine, Taurine, Arginine

Water-Soluble Vitamins
Vitamins C, B1, B3, B6, B12,
Folate, Choline,
Pantothenic acid

Essential Fatty Acids
Docosahexanoic acid (DHA)
Eicosapentanoic acid (EPA)
Gamma linoleic acid (GLA)

Minerals
Calcium, Potassium,
Magnesium

Others
Coenzyme Q10, Bromelain,
Lecithin, Glucomannan,
Pycnogenol, Beta Carotene,

Herbs
Cayenne, Ginger,
Hawthorn, Garlic

Trimethylglycine (Betaine),
Grape Seed Extract,
Wine Phytonutrients

get severe enough, the artery cannot adequately deliver blood and its associated oxygen and nutrients to the target site. Subsequently, the site suffers from the deficit, whether it's the heart, skeletal muscles, kidneys, brain or wherever. Such suffering may manifest itself as pain, limited stamina, mental deficits or decreased organ function of various types.

If the blockage gets bad enough, the target tissue dies. When that happens to the brain, it's a form of a stroke. In the heart muscle, it's a heart attack.

Sometimes these deposits (atheromas) trap calcium and other minerals within them, causing a hardening of the artery (calcific sclerosis). However, this is more or less an academic issue at our level. Quite simply, we don't want that stuff getting into our blood vessels, hard or soft. If it's already there, we want it gone!

Certainly a desirable goal, but is it feasible? We know the situation is preventable; our ancestors did it consistently, and for a long period of time, until fairly recently. But, is it reversible?

Current Treatment Methods

Conventional medicine's approach to this problem has been predictable: treat symptoms and cut out, bypass, or stretch diseased areas. Besides the invasiveness and cost, this philosophy presents the additional dilemma of not dealing with the cause or causes. And, what do you do when too many areas are affected to invasively treat them all?

Now it even appears that these short term, quick fix techniques have a less-than-stellar track record by almost any standard. As far back as 1983 the People's Medical Society reported that coronary bypass surgeries, which were growing at an amazing rate, were not preventing heart attacks. Further, the *New England Journal of Medicine* (May 6, 1982) was quoted as saying that "only 15 percent of patients who survive a myocardial infarction are likely to have their lives prolonged by surgery."

Concerning angina (the pain associated with low blood flow to heart muscle), the *Journal of the American Medical Association* (*JAMA*, Feb. 13, 1981) was quoted as saying, "Angina will recur or progress after bypass surgery in about five percent of patients per year." The explanation for this was tied to the finding that about 20 percent of the surgical grafts clog up within twelve months of surgery, with the percentage rising each succeeding year.

What's even more bizarre is that there was no difference in survival rates back then between heart surgery and medical (drug) treatment. This was still true as of May 1997, when the *New England Journal of Medicine* reported on a study between Canadian and American heart patients and their subsequent death rates after a heart attack. About eight times the percentage of Americans as their Canadian counterparts received either bypass surgery or angioplasty (surgical attempts to open arteries). At the end of one year following the heart attack, the death rate was the same in both groups. *JAMA*, in November, 1992 (v 268, #18), had already said that an estimated 50 percent of the tests being done to diagnose serious heart disease (coronary angiography) were "unnecessary, or at least could be postponed."

It seems to me that the quick fix may not be the answer. A lifestyle change is in order if you really want to alter outcomes.

Be careful if you think pharmaceuticals are the answer. They may be, but it's hard to say. In 1995, a study found that the six million people who were taking a popular class of drug to control blood pressure (calcium channel blockers) may actually be increasing their chance of having a heart attack. This came after previous studies showing concern over use of the drugs right after a heart attack or to prevent a second one.

Ah, but fear not; the all-too-conventional American Heart Association (AHA) has entered the dietary arena, with foods that are "heart healthy." Robert Atkins, M.D., proponent of a high-protein, low-carbohydrate diet lifestyle, described in his *Health Revelations* newsletter (December 1997) the technique for gaining endorsement of a food product by this organization. It seems that if your product is low in fat, saturated fat, and cholesterol, that's all it takes. That's it. Of course, that's with the exception of a $2,500 one-time fee, and an annual renewable fee of $650. Dr. Atkins notes, almost comically (though it's anything but comical) that Pop Tarts and jelly beans qualify! (This sort of reminds me of the time I found the words "a low-fat food" printed on the label of a chocolate-coated peppermint candy bar—no kidding.)

Most of us have heard that butter is bad for us (though it's been in use for thousands of years), and that margarine is the way to go for heart health. Again (broken record here), you have to be careful messing with new age, quick fixes to problems that may not be there. In 1995, a shocking study came out following several previous ones showing margarine isn't all we've been told. A report by a Harvard Medical School epidemiologist (of 865 Framingham Study participants) showed that those using margarine had twice the heart disease risk over those who didn't. What's more, the "evil" butter was found to cause no harm. And now we have newer, synthetic, miracle fats that aren't even absorbed!

Another piece of "news" we've heard for years is how bad salt is for us, especially as a cardiovascular stress with its ability to increase blood pressure. It ends up that even this issue is not as cut and dried as we've been led to believe. Evidence has now emerged (in an obviously controversial study) that the less salt people eat, the higher the risk of experiencing untimely death! Dr. Michael Alderman, chairman of epidemiology at the Albert Einstein School of Medicine, and president of the American Society of Hypertension, headed the study that stated, among other things, "It is possible that the harm of a low-sodium diet may outweigh its benefit. The lower the sodium, the worse off you are" (Ross 1998).

Two months later, the *Journal of the American Medical Association* published a related report, concluded the following: "These results do not support a general recommendation to reduce sodium intake" (Graudal 1998).

I personally am not in favor of going overboard on the salt. However, there is an important issue here that is often missed. Most of the salt we use is refined salt with important minerals removed. In fact, I believe our craving for salt is due to our need for many of these minerals, especially magnesium. The problem is, these minerals are worth a lot of money if sold independently, so they are removed before we're sold the remaining pure sodium chloride product. Even most "sea salt" has been through a similar process. Though from the sea, once the minerals are removed it's just not worth the extra price.

The exception, of course, would be natural salt that does not have any minerals removed. This may be less of a problem in countries other than the U.S., but I can so far only find two companies in the States that offer true, unrefined salt for human consumption:

> The Grain & Salt Society, Inc.
> 273 Fairway Drive
> Asheville, North Carolina 28805
> 800-TOP-SALT (867-7258), 828-299-9005
> www.celtic-seasalt.com

> Redmond Minerals, Inc.
> P.O. Box 219
> Redmond, Utah 84652
> 800-367-7258, 435-529-7402
> www.realsalt.com

We've discussed refined sugar, refined flour and artificial non-foods. Now think of their prevalence in our diet. We've mentioned the possible damage by our chlorinated city water (and homogenized milk) on arterial walls, and how the body defends itself with cholesterol, instead of the substance itself being the problem.

Small wonder our killer disease remains number one.

What Can You Do?

Besides the general plan in Chapter 20, there's much you can do specifically, with research behind it (though poorly publicized), to obtain that heart health insurance policy.

The nutrients to concentrate on, in my opinion (and while you do your own research to find what you think may be best for you), are in two small groups. The first I call the CCME group, and the second is the homocysteine group.

CCME was first coined by Brian Leibovitz, Ph.D., of the Institute for the Study of Optimal Nutrition in the institute's *Journal of Optimal Nutrition* (3(3), 1994), and stands for L-carnitine, coenzyme Q10, magnesium and vitamin E. He is quick to say that this emphasis should not diminish the importance of the other factors, only that these have an established role in the all-important role of energy production. To quote Dr. Leibovitz, "Carnitine carries fats across the inner membrane for beta-oxidation. Coenzyme Q10 is the key factor in the electron transport system. Magnesium is an essential cofactor for many of the enzyme sys-

---

The Suggested Preventive Daily Doses for CCME

For a 154-pound (70-kg) adult

L-Carnitine:	1,000 mg
Coenzyme Q10:	100 mg
Magnesium:	500 to 800 mg
Vitamin E: (as mixed tocopherols)	400 to 800 IU

tems that support energy production. Vitamin E is in the membrane where it can scavenge the free radicals generated by the electron transport system."

That's as technical as we're going to get. Suffice it to say they have important roles in supplying energy to the heart muscle (and others) for proper functioning.

(For the more aggressive enthusiast, the amino acid taurine has been shown it can be as effective as coenzyme Q10 for cardiac output, congestive heart failure, edema (swelling) and palpitations. This was in the *Japanese Circulation Journal*, vol. 56, Jan. 1992. However, 3 grams per day may be necessary for effect, and it's better taken between meals for best absorption.)

The homocysteine group is the brainchild of Dr. Kilmer McCully, a Harvard physician who published his theory back in 1969, explaining that excess homocysteine in the blood causes vastly increased risks of heart disease. Instead of the Nobel Prize for Medicine, he was denied tenure. He subsequently found (and was independently confirmed) that increases as little as 12 percent over average can more than triple a man's heart attack risk. Ironically, the confirmation study came from Harvard; it just happened to be over twenty years late (1992 data published from *The Physicians' Health Study*). Public acclaim has finally been given to this man, which he richly deserves.

The mechanism involves the deficiency of an enzyme that properly breaks down an amino acid, methionine. When this deficiency develops, methionine generates a by-product called homocysteine, which then accumulates (and can be measured in the blood). The higher it goes, the higher the risk of heart disease. What's neat is that this increase can be quickly brought down, using nutrient therapy. Though there are two other agents that can also do the trick (choline, trimethylglycine), the cheapest and most readily available are the vitamins B6, B12 and folic acid.

So, the general plan in Chapter 20 may by itself offer the protective influence you need to lower serum homocysteine levels, as all are in the multivitamin suggested. For additional protection, especially if you are considered high risk for heart disease (see your doc), you can consider the following:

- 1,000 micrograms of vitamin B12, sublingual (SL) form, one/week: As oral forms may not be well absorbed, the SL form is preferable, unless you have access to injectable (and happen to prefer it!).
- Folic acid, 800 micrograms/day: It's hard to get more in the U.S., though it's available in much higher doses in other countries. It's limited to avoid a nerve degeneration problem by masking a deficiency of vitamin B12—sort of a nonproblem, as long as you take B12, which most everyone admits is about as nontoxic as anything gets.
- Vitamin B6, 50 milligrams/day: There is popular propaganda that B6 can cause nerve damage, but it takes over 500 milligrams, and usually more, every day for months to encounter this in anyone with normal function (and they improve once it's discontinued). Occurrences are very rare, and too little B6 presents the same symptoms! Why aren't we warned of permanent drug damage problems with the same fervor, like liver with acetaminophen, or stomach with aspirin?

I fear there are a lot of politics (and economics) in many of the answers throughout this book, but we'll leave that for others to deal with. Right now our goal is to get healthy and stay there!

Chelation Therapy: A Faster Option

For those already diagnosed with cardiovascular disease, and who may need a faster, "jump-start" technique, there is another tool available to you. It does not involve surgery and can get into all arteries with its effect. It has a long history of both safety and efficacy, and rarely, if ever, are we told about it.

It's chelation therapy, or intravenous EDTA, which stands for ethylene-diamine-tetra-acetic acid, administered by a solution into a vein. This remarkable treatment has been given, in dozens of doses, to thousands of people, and is probably offered near where you live.

EDTA is a chelating agent, meaning it grabs onto different molecules in the blood, allowing the body to eliminate them in the urine. Calcium is one of the minerals removed, and the idea is this agent pulls it out of blood vessel walls to help break down arterial plaque material. It seems to preferentially take abnormal deposits first, but nutritional supplements are given anyway during treatment, so that the body can replace those removed.

As some of the patients getting the therapy are pretty sick, the kidneys must be allowed adequate time to remove the minerals. This mandates sessions lasting about three hours each time, which is usually spent lying around in lounge chairs reading, watching TV, or talking to the other recipients. How quickly the treatment can be repeated depends on how good the kidney status is. Usually this can be up to three times per week, depending on the person's health. Monitoring of the status is performed using laboratory testing, and the whole procedure has stringent protocols put forth by the American College of Advancement in Medicine (ACAM).

A series of treatments is usually around thirty sessions, and some people get maintenance sessions at intervals afterward. Cost is around $120 per treatment, so a whole series is far less than a single surgery, and more insurance companies are starting to handle them.

For more information on this modality, contact ACAM, at 800-532-3688.

CHAPTER 16

Elimination of Constipation

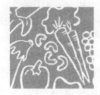

FUN TOPIC. Unfortunately, not a funny topic, neither an insignificant one. Everybody knows someone who is haunted with the problem of constipation, or they have been constipated themselves at one time or another. What many people do not know is that constipation is totally abnormal, always, and abnormal enough that with the exception of those unlucky souls with serious medical syndromes or surgical interventions, nearly everyone with this problem can effect a huge difference in their regularity without taking medications of any kind.

Any remaining exceptions are those who just don't care (they probably aren't reading this), and some who have been on drugs for the situation for so many years that the body has developed a tolerance to them (which it does). Even those can be handled with herbs that are gentler than the pharmaceuticals we see daily on television.

The importance of nontoxic, nutritional treatment for constipation is significant. The problem is a lot more serious than just a snicker over the dinner table or taking an occasional laxative. It can be a chronic nightmare, and it may very well be an indicator of more trouble to come.

So Just What's the Big Deal?

I was taught in medical school that the colon was not an absorptive organ; that is, the small intestine did the absorbing of nutrients and "stuff," and the colon, or large intestine, just pulled the water out, firming up what's left for the big moment.

I don't buy it. I didn't then, and I certainly don't now.

If the colon does not absorb things other than water, why are there so many medications that use the rectal, or suppository, route of administration? To the body, most medications are toxins, due to the fact that they are designed to overrule a process in the body and force something to happen that wasn't happening by itself. It may be something desirable, but it forces it nonetheless. Why else would we use them? (Not that they aren't useful—many of them are).

The point is, they are not nutrients, and they are absorbed.

The stool is packed with the "undesirables" of the diet (except for undigestible fiber; that's desirable). Anything solid the body doesn't want, it tries to excrete in the stool, and if the colon can absorb non-native chemicals, it can absorb other "stuff" in the stool that the body might prefer to do without, if it could get rid of it quickly enough.

What's worse, like any decaying material, the stool contains things that putrefy *(rot)*, and others that either ferment or can go rancid. Wouldn't it be more desirable to have such neat little processes occurring in the sewer, instead of the bowel? Could a constipated person's bowel be turning into a sewer, with all the diseases and undesirable organisms that turn up there?

Could that be one reason a lot of us don't feel good?

I suppose that it would be appropriate to establish just what constipation is in the first place. How long does it take for a person to become constipated? Two weeks? If you have a bowel movement every other day, without exception, and you never need laxatives of any kind for such bowel habits, could you still be having a problem with constipation?

Both *Dorland's Medical Dictionary* and the *Merck Manual of Diagnosis and Therapy* define "constipation" as bowel movements that are "infrequent" and "difficult." It is not uncommon to find medical texts that say *three bowel movements per week* is normal!

I have to take exception to that.

This medical description of regularity makes sense in that it is an accurate depiction of the average bowel habits in America today. Today's average, however, does not necessarily mean that it's normal.

In days past (way past), when fiber remained intact in our food and our fluid intake was not only greater, but also consisted of more water, stools were passed at least once a day, and less was considered abnormal, simply because that's what was considered the norm. In my opinion, really normal bowel habits means twice per day, with one daily as the outside limit. (Nutritionists who study daily habits of "backward" cultures, having totally natural diets, report that a movement after each meal is the norm.)

The modern diet is responsible for this change in definition. As we refine our foods more and more, then increase our intake of those altered staples (sugar, flour, bread, pasta, etc.) the problem begins. Even the current food pyramid has grain products as the base of the pyramid, meaning that those foods are the ones that should be eaten most. Ignoring whether that should really be the case in our diet, the real significance is that rarely are the flours, the breads, the pastas, the cereals, or the grains (rice, barley, etc.) available as 100 percent whole-grain products. One of the first things to leave during processing, in a high amount, is the natural fiber that the whole food contained.

That fiber was meant to be a partner in a normal process constantly at work in our gastrointestinal (GI) tract called "peristalsis." This is a wavelike contraction and relaxation motion that travels along the bowel wall moving ingested material through the intestinal tract until it is expelled out the bottom end. Normal amounts of fiber, along with adequate fluids, permit this motion to more efficiently "grab" the bowel contents and move them along that all-important path.

With the "stuff" in the bowel now remaining in there longer than by original design, the putrefying, fermenting, decaying, etc., mentioned earlier have more time to occur (and cause symptoms). However, there's more to it than that. The bowel seems to "know" that those contents aren't supposed to be in there too long, so it tries harder to evacuate them. In so doing, it applies greater pressures along the gut wall in an effort to get the job done.

Unfortunately, such an undertaking is not without its consequences. A chain is as strong as its weakest link and, like old-fashioned inner tubes, the bowel wall has weaker and stronger areas. With the increased pressure, a weak area can stretch and balloon out, causing a small pocket to form (or many of them, in fact), branching out sideways from the main flow through the intestine. These pouches are called diverticuli, and the situation is called diverticulosis. When the pouches become inflamed, from trapped material festering there, this is called diverticulitis, which can be very painful. This isn't news to too many people.

The same abnormal pressure situation is responsible, farther down, for not permitting normal blood return through veins surrounding the rectal area. The blood backs up, stretching the vessels through which it flows, and in time becomes noticeable as hemorrhoids, which are varicose veins localized to this area. These, too, are not particularly pleasant. They are, however, as well as the diverticuli (and regular varicose veins, which can also be caused by constipation), more easily prevented than eradicated, so handling constipation before such situations manifest themselves can pay rich dividends in terms of hassles avoided.

In addition to diverticulosis, hemorrhoids, and varicose veins, constipation can also cause headaches, insomnia, gas problems, indigestion, and even cancer.

So, What to Do?

The first fix is simple, if not altogether easy: Do your best to avoid any products made with refined flour. (Does this sound familiar? If not, head back to Chapter 3.) This would include the same flour, bread, pasta, pastries, cookies, rolls, muffins, bagels, rice, corn and other grains we've mentioned before.

You'll notice that the answers repeat themselves because the questions are really the same; bad health in our "civilized" world is due in large part to the same common mistakes we make every day in overlooking the dangers that confront us in our daily diet. Also, remember that refined sugar has all the fiber removed (Chapter 2). You, of course, can take fiber supplements, but remember that many have artificial sweeteners aboard, and it's possible to take enough that vitamins can be bound up in the fiber and inadequately absorbed. I prefer to do it with food, but it's obviously an option. (Drink liquids fairly heavily when on fiber supplements.)

Water's right up there again, too. Good water. You don't have to be waterlogged to get the job done, but you should be drinking enough good water to go slightly beyond the satisfaction of thirst. If this doesn't sound familiar then take another look at Chapter 4.

Other Causes

There are a few other things besides congenital and surgical situations that can cause constipation. Iron supplements are known to do that, as well as pharmaceuticals such as antidepressants and some pain medications. Read labels carefully, looking for side effects that include constipation.

As you might remember from Chapter 6, antibiotics can alter the intestinal environment sufficiently to affect normal function in the gut. Probiotics (acidophilus) can be noticeably helpful, even by itself, in helping with constipation. One quarter to one half teaspoon before meals and bedtime for just a few days has made a difference in those with low or altered gut flora as a predisposing factor.

Low thyroid function can cause constipation. If your blood tests are normal, but you have cold hands and feet, are tired or sluggish all the time, and gain weight easily (along with constipation), it could still be involved. Consider temperature testing at home, as per Broda Barnes' book, *Hypothyroidism: The Unsuspected Illness,* or *Solved: The Riddle of Illness,* by Langer & Scheer.

If your constipation is relatively new, and you haven't done anything you can think of as a possible cause, a visit to your doctor might be in order to rule out any medical explanation in or around the GI tract. A barium enema, an un-fun, but not excruciating x-ray test, can give a good picture of the bowel and may be used in the workup. Though a fair amount of x-ray is utilized in the test, it does show the area pretty well. Endoscopy (inserting a fiberoptic tube up from below to allow true visualization of the bowel's inner surface) may also be used, but cannot get as far up as the barium test. These modalities can find masses, inflammations, and other problems that could be involved in constipation.

Allergies can alter peristalsis, so a search for food sensitivities is appropriate. Wheat, milk, corn, and soy are right at the top of the list, followed by peanut, egg, and any type of artificial color, flavor, enhancer, preservative, etc., that the body may not be used to (as per Chapter 5). It's also worth looking at foods that are craved or eaten every day. That by itself puts that food high on the "suspect" list until proven otherwise.

Confirming food allergies cannot be done with the standard skin "prick" testing. There are blood tests, such as RAST (radioallergosorbent test), that can help, but they are not infallible. See the lab list in the back if you want to seek further help in this area. Probably the best test for this is cytotoxic testing, but it's very hard to find.

The standard, and cheapest, suggestion is to avoid the suspect food for seven days (twenty-one days for dairy). That means TOTAL abstinence, or the test period starts over. Then you can reintroduce the suspect item and see if symptoms occur . . . any symptoms. If you feel worse during the first few days of the test, the chances are greater that the suspect food is involved, and also greater that you'll feel better at the end of the test period.

It's possible that you can be allergic to milk, but not to cream, or cheese, or yogurt, etc. You just have to be patient, analyze and learn about your body, and keep looking. It's also possible that, after quitting an allergic food, you can get it back on a limited basis, where once per week, say, does not cause symptoms, while twice per week does.

A final food manipulation is the old standby, and it really works: prunes. You can, most likely, find a number of these handy, tasty little items that will handle your constipation. Avoid those treated with sulfur dioxide or sugar.

For those in whom dietary manipulation and acidophilus are

inadequate, there are a few other things to try. I have found that a trial of digestive enzymes can, in some people, be very helpful. I usually use Super Enzyme, by Twinlab, two right after meals (see Appendix).

For quick relief, medication still is most likely unnecessary. Magnesium capsules, of any type, available at any health food store, are the closest thing to "dial-a-stool" I've ever seen. Starting with a 500 milligram capsule at bedtime, and increasing by one capsule each night, you can find a dose that causes any stage desired, from slightly soft, to loose, to downright get outta the way.

Vitamin C in high enough doses, will loosen the stools. I like this idea because it also is a detoxifier at the same time, and few people receive enough of this marvelous nutrient anyway (see Chapter 9). However, it requires a lot of capsules, usually, to reach bowel tolerance (the point where the stools loosen), and many people are reticent to swallow so many supplements if they aren't used to nutrient therapies, so I save this option for those a bit more enlightened (and most of those don't have constipation problems anyway).

You may find what are called homeopathic remedies for constipation in the health food store. These can be effective and are nontoxic. (See Chapter 12.)

Finally, a well-known herb for constipation is cascara sagrada. This can be very effective, so read labels carefully and start at a low dose. The least that works is the best.

CHAPTER 17

The In's and Out's of Healthy Skin

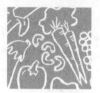

HEALTHY SKIN. We all want it; however, some are willing to work harder for it than others. For those who don't have the time to spend all day pampering their skin (which might be the wrong way, wasting tons of time or even doing damage), these are the basic "in's and out's" of rewarding skin care.

Bear in mind, I mean the term "in's and out's" literally. I firmly believe, through personal observation and research, that skin can be clearly (pun intented) affected by things we do both ways—applications to the skin's surface (out's) and by oral nutrition (in's). Anyone who believes otherwise just hasn't tried or maybe hasn't tried correctly.

What About the "Out" Theory?

Skeptics of the "out" theory may doubt there really is something you can put on your skin to actually make a difference in how it looks, at least over the long haul. I would ask them to remember several points of interest. First, the skin is not only a body organ in its own right, but it's also the largest organ of the body. It obviously has healing and regenerative powers of remarkable degree, or cuts, bruises, scratches, abrasions, etc., would never get better.

Statistically, there is little question that antibiotic ointments lessen superficial skin infections (though I'm not saying they are the best ointments available). Rashes improve with cortisone creams, itching decreases with antihistamine lotions, and even hemorrhoids shrink with the right topical preparation. Conversely, allergens can inflame the skin on contact, and topical toxins can do even worse damage.

Whether a doubter or not, for those open minded enough to at least try a few things, let's start with the "out's," and discuss some topical applications that might show some results. These effects tend to occur a bit faster than the "in's," since most (though not all) internally controlled changes start at the basal layer of skin, which is many cell layers removed from the surface. This means improvements will not really be visible until the change has been incorporated into the cells reaching the surface. Anyway, from the outside, here are a few ideas, starting with what not to apply, which can be as important as what to apply.

What *Not* to Apply to Your Skin

- *Avoid mineral oil.* Avoid it like the plague! Read labels and buy nothing that contains it. A travesty perpetrated on children is to call that stuff "baby oil." This is a great way to stress and age skin. Mineral oil is very cheap and is readily absorbed into the skin, which is why it's used, as most people want something that goes in fast and are willing to fall for a company's advertising propaganda that a product is high quality.

  Plus, mineral oil gives the skin a really nice glow—for a while. Though absorbed, the stuff is poorly assimilated (if at all), so it sits within the skin, merrily damaging the vitamin D apparatus of the body, while your body has to work at a way to detoxify and remove it. This makes your skin age. (By the way, the proper source of vitamin D is the skin, not that white stuff we call pasteurized, homogenized, vitamin D-enriched cow's milk.)

There are magnificent substitutes for mineral oil. They are vegetable based, including light vitamin E, safflower, almond, and other cold-pressed, unrefined oils. Again, you are probably stuck visiting a good health food store or dedicated natural health supplier.

• *Avoid deodorant soaps and germicidal cleansers.* The skin absorbs stuff! If you can't pronounce it, keep it off your skin. Some of you may remember the controversy over a skin cleanser containing hexachlorophene, later only available by prescription when it was discovered that the chemical had toxic side effects and was absorbed into the skin too easily. For the same reason you have to respect the lotions used for kids who have head lice, etc. (Read those labels sometime!) With chemicals, you must respect and baby your skin.

• *Avoid excessive makeup, especially heavy base coats.* Skin pores need to be open to air as much as possible, to expel sebum, toxins, sweat, etc. The least amount of makeup is the best, and absolutely never leave it on overnight. The water-based products are the least occlusive to pores as a rule, and the best are usually found under less-known health store brands, rather than huge Madison Avenue logos (though this is changing). Also, look out for mineral oil in many make-up products.

• *Avoid excessive suntanning.* (See #2 under "What to Apply to Your Skin.")

• *Avoid tanning booths.* This is not the same as sunlight and don't forget it. You have a different spectrum of light here, and it's not nice to fool Mother Nature.

• *Avoid washing too soon after suntanning.* After getting some sun, the oils on your skin are beneficial to the vitamin D mechanism, so try to leave them on for an hour or so before washing them off.

What to Apply to Your Skin

• *Apply a little sun.* Please note the operative word is a little, not enough to deep fry and charbroil. Ten or fifteen minutes, both sides, allows natural sun rays to bathe and stimulate the skin, generating vitamin D without doing damage.

• *Use only the highest-quality moisturizing or suntanning lotions.* How do you find these? You are pretty much restricted to good health food stores or skin-care companies that really care. Two national companies that have done their homework are Nature's Gate and Mill Creek. Where I'm from we have a good regional brand called Trader Joe's.

What might be called one of the "ultimate" skin lotions (also available as a cream), is called Rejuvenex, by Life Extension (www.lef.org, 800-544-4440, 954-766-8433). I'm not sure why users are so enthusiastic about this product, but many are. It's more expensive than most standard skin preparations. You'll have to decide for yourself whether it's worth it.

Read labels! Besides avoiding mineral oil, you want the largest list of ingredients with a history of being beneficial for the skin, such as vitamin E (tocopherol), vitamin A (retinoids), wheat germ oil, rosemary, tea tree oil, aloe vera, sesame oil, jojoba and many others. Though this isn't an absolute guarantee, the fact that a company even bothered to find and add small amounts of so many "thought-to-be-good-for-the-skin" nutrients is usually a decided plus.

• *Loofah-type skin stimulation.* This is where you don't want to be too gentle. A loofah, for the uninitiated, is a natural type of sponge that feels sort of rough. It helps remove dead skin cells, and it opens pores. You don't want to cause abrasions, of course, but moderate stimulation of the skin can be beneficial, especially when done on a daily basis. (It also helps awaken you in the morning.) Be more gentle on the face, and in bad cases of cystic acne, go really easy or avoid it altogether.

• *Aalpha hydroxy acids (AHAs).* This is a major subject area in its own right, since it reentered the cosmetic scene in the late 1970s. (The ancient Romans and the ancient Egyptians before them, including Cleopatra, beat you to it.) Though mostly manufactured synthetically now (only citric and lactic acids are reliably natural), these are also called "fruit acids," due to their natural origins.

AHAs dissolve the intercellular "cement" that holds more superficial skin cells together, opening pores and uncovering smoother, deeper skin layers. This explanation apparently is a bit simplistic because research has found other skin benefits that cannot be fully ascribed to it alone.

AHAs are useful in both dry and oily skin types, both young and old skin, and both postpubertal and postmenopausal skin problems. Since side effects began appearing from some of the non-AHA prescription exfoliative skin products, the fruit acids have really taken off. (There are prescription strengths of AHAs also, but we're basically talking about over-the-counter products here.)

A bit too fantastic? Maybe, but read all you can find on the subject before you write it off. You may be missing a very big boat. If you decide to give AHAs a try, I might recommend a buffered product in the neighborhood of 10 percent, except around sensitive areas like eyes, neck, and upper chest, where lower concentrations are more appropriate. Apply to dry skin only (moist skin absorbs better and may be more susceptible to irritation), and start slow, at least until you know exactly how you react (there is often a tingling sensation at first, but this is rarely sensitizing—unlike some prescription, non-AHA agents.)

The originally patented AHA, glycolic acid, is still my preference. It has the most research behind it and is the smallest molecule, so it can go deeper. But there are many excellent products available of all sorts of AHAs. (There are also poorer ones, and price is not always the deciding factor, so speak with a skin-care expert you trust before spending too much money here.) Properly selected and utilized, you may be truly amazed at what the fruit acids can do for you.

That's the basics, from the outside. Now let's briefly get just a bit more specific.

The topic of skin fills whole sections of medical school libraries, so we have to be selective. There are two skin care problems that we should address, without having to deal with actual skin diseases. One situation is puberty, and the other is postmenopause. These often are times of unique symptoms, but ones which may be considerably helped without major medical intervention. We'll deal with each as additions to the basic recommendations.

Puberty

The first is puberty, a time of wild changes in hormonal outputs for both sexes. Though this can be an exciting time for most, the havoc that can be wreaked upon the skin is less than desirable. Excessive oils are produced, and blockages with subsequent inflammation of pores occur, among other things. (What kids do with food from the inside has no small effect, for sure, but let's deal with the "outs.") Assuming you're one of those with adolescent skin problems, what can one do, topically, before heading for the prescription drugs?

• **Benzoyl peroxide.** This is one over-the-counter medication that really can help. Besides being a simple cleanser and providing some beneficial stimulation for blood flow to problem areas, peroxide has other advantages: it supplies oxygenation to pores, it has the ability to work its way deeper than superficial scrubbing can reach, and it is strong enough to kill many bacteria. The bubbling of peroxide in skin wounds can work its way into the tracts of abscesses and even fistulae (longer, deeper tracts). This is the only acceptable germicide, as its action is only with oxygen.

• **Vitamin E oil/Vitamin A oil rotations.** This one sounds crazy, but hear me out. Though oily skin may haunt the hapless teenager, applying the right oils to the skin can not only nourish it, but also lessen the body's desire (need/ability) to manufacture its own.

Here's what you do. At night, before retiring, take a capsule of vitamin E oil and puncture it. Apply the oil to the face, and leave it on overnight, washing it off in the morning. The next night, do the same thing with a capsule of vitamin A oil. Use a pillow case you don't mind ruining and try to ignore the odor of vitamin A. Since everything is removed in the morning, no one even knows you're doing something "weird," and the results often can be seen within one to two weeks, so you don't have to do it forever to see if you are going to be one of the lucky ones. If you notice any benefit, lessen the frequency to the least that works to maintain the gains, and then experiment to see which oil is the the more helpful for you. (One oil is usually superior to the other, but it can vary depending on the person.)

One last point here. The prescription vitamin A-acid preparations are derivations of the vitamin A part of this technique. They are incredibly more expensive, and they are riddled with side effects, while you are led to believe that the natural source either doesn't work, or is too toxic!

Postmenopause

Now, what about menopause, and the postmenopausal period? There are many misconceptions about estrogen and progesterone, including their effects on skin, bones and cancer, along with physical symptoms they can cause, especially when internal production of each decreases. (Even testosterone in women can be involved.)

As far as skin is concerned, progesterone is worth discussing: First and foremost, don't panic. Many who have been on progesterone and experienced side effects haven't really been on true progesterone at all. Almost all prescription medications called progesterone, whether used orally, as a patch, topically, or otherwise, are progestins, meaning they are synthetically changed molecules similar to natural progesterone but different enough to be patentable. (That's where the money is. You didn't think they were changing molecules for *your* benefit, did you?)

The problems with the non-natural progestins, besides being expensive, are that they don't do all the jobs progesterone was supposed to do while causing side effects at the same time.

Natural progesterone, on the other hand, has no side effects, as long as you don't take so much that you cause your period to start again. (Wouldn't that be fun.) Long before that happens, not only do most women feel better, but also their skin holds moisture better (more youthful appearing) over time, bruises less, and handles all trauma better. Now, how do you get and use the right stuff?

Natural progesterone as a cream is a bit tough to find, but its immediate precursor is more readily available. The problem is you want active hormone, which requires a chemical conversion. Look for labels that contain actual progesterone. Most good health food stores have it as Mexican yam cream, under multiple brand names. One popular one is Progest™.

Probably the strongest available nonprescription product can be located by calling Life Extension Foundation, an excellent company that carries a multitude of hard-to-find health products. Theirs is supposed to be already converted to the real thing, which would be an advantage if for some reason your body were a poor converter. (Purchased items are at a discount if you are a member.) Their number is 800-841-5433. (Natural progesterone cream is available by prescription. It needs a compounding pharmacist, and a doctor enlightened enough to know where to order it.)

Once you've found the stuff, use it twice a day, approximately 1/4 to 1/2 teaspoon per application, for about three weeks on, then one week off. It is applied to soft areas of skin on a rotating basis because after several days the local skin cells saturate with it, and it becomes harder to rub in. Just move to a different area, such as face, breasts, abdomen, and inner arms and legs for a few days. Hands, feet, and outer (thicker-skinned) arm/leg areas are less desirable. Even vaginal applications are fine.

Local use is distributed system wide to the whole body, but rotate use to the face when possible, because the rewards of a potent moisturizer may be most obvious here. A great discussion on progesterone (along with other hormones for postmenopausal women) is contained in the excellent book, *Natural Hormone Replacement*, by Wright & Morgenthaler. The book can be ordered at 800-543-3873; 707-769-8016 (F); www.smart-publications.com.

The Inside

Okay. You've played all the games with your skin from the outside. Whether the results were great or were limited, there is more you can do—a lot more. Now the car is painted and waxed, but the octane of the fuel is what makes the big difference. (The difference with the car analogy is that good fuel to the body is used everywhere, including the skin.)

There are more doubters, I believe, of the "in" theory. How can foods and supplements have anything to do with how good your skin looks on the surface? This leads to the fundamental question of whether we even need additional vitamins or other nutrients at all. I deal with this subject at length in Chapter 6. These same skeptics admit to the use of oral antibiotics for skin lesions, oral steroids for rashes, and oral doses of antihistamines for itching. Ingestion of various substances affects the skin. Don't believe for a second that foods and supplements can't also have an effect (both good and bad).

Let's take a look at what can be done, both what you should and shouldn't do, from the inside out to protect your body's most visible organ.

Things to Avoid

In a civilized world, there are tons of things that should be avoided, actually, but we'll concentrate on those with the best chances of having a direct effect on the skin that you might see as an improvement over the ensuing weeks.

• *Avoid all types of white or refined sugar.* Sugar is concentrated to a point that the body does not handle it as nutritious food, but as a body stress, both on the pancreas and the immune system. (White cells, the "cleaner-uppers" of debris and infection in the body, respond slower when challenged with concentrated sugar.) Also, sugar uses up the zinc in the tissues, which is vital for healthy skin.

- *Avoid chocolate.* You can always find someone ready to tell you there is no problem here, but the teenage crowd, as a rule, is definitely affected. Not only is it wall-to-wall sugar, but also it is an adrenal stress, even if the individual is not sensitive to it.

- *Avoid fried foods.* These use terrible oils. Once heated, they are chemically changed and should not be in the body. Their effect on oily skin can be pronounced. The problem is not eating fat; it's what kind of fat. Fresh, unprocessed, cold-pressed oils are okay, just hard to find. (Wok frying, if you do it quickly, is acceptable.)

- *Avoid craved foods.* At least check them by not eating them for a week. You may be sensitive to foods that you crave, and the skin may show the effects. If you give up a food for a week and you feel worse for the first few days, you should be highly suspicious of that food item.

- *Avoid antibiotics, especially the long term ones.* Tetracyclines, erythromycins, etc., do not get to the cause of skin problems, which stems from the body's response to bacteria and not the bacteria themselves. This is why discontinuing the drug is often accompanied by more acne. Especially noteworthy is the possibility of overgrowth of yeasts and fungi with antibiotic use, since these organisms are totally immune to the mode of action of these drugs.

Things to Do

Now, what are some of the things to do for the inside to nourish the skin? Keep in mind that many nutritional changes for skin can take up to three months to see because the fat-soluble vitamins may be involved. Since they are incorporated into the deepest layer of skin first (the germinal layer), they must grow into each progressively higher layer as the outermost layers slough off.

- **A good multivitamin.** This is a must, to tie everything together. By "good," I mean one that is stronger than the U.S. Recommended Dietary Allowances (RDA). (Anyone who says the RDA is adequate must not have tried higher doses or is just unaware of current nutritional studies.) To find a good multivitamin, look on the list of amounts on the label. Usually, there is an area with vitamins B1, B2, and B6 together. Find it, and if each one lists a strength of 25 mg (milligrams) or more, the product is a strong one. For example, an excellent start is Multi-Energy™ by Solaray™. Get the one that does not contain iron, and take it twice a day.

- **Zinc.** This is taken in addition to whatever is contained in the multivitamin, about 50 mg per day in the chelated form or as zinc picolinate. Don't get carried away because high doses can cause deficiencies in copper, though I do not believe this is common. Zinc and vitamin A are powerful nutrients for skin and work well together.

- **Vitamin A.** This works better for skin as real vitamin A, not beta carotene (its precursor), since beta-carotene is not fat soluble. There are all sorts of tales about the toxicity of vitamin A, but I find it vastly easier to be deficient. Stay with natural fish oil A (no synthetics), and 10,000 to 25,000 IU (international units) is a reasonable maintenance dose for skin. (Check with your doctor if you think you are having side effects, and avoid it if you are using prescription vitamin A acid preparations of any type or are trying to get pregnant.)

  In my practice, I found that an initial daily dose of at least 50,000 IU was necessary for about three months before considering maintenance doses. (For the record, from 600 to 800 deaths per year are reported as caused by aspirin, while the death rate from natural vitamin A supplements is zero for the past fifty years.)

- **Vitamin C.** This is a major component in the manufacture of collagen, which is the number one repair protein in the body, including skin. It also helps protect against all sorts of toxicities, but the RDA is nowhere near enough. I would recommend 1,000 mg, two times per day. As you should know by now, don't bother with time-release types, and capsules are better than hard pills. If you have any trouble tolerating it, you can switch from ascorbic acid to an ascorbate, which does not bother the stomach.

For the Puberty Group, I Might Add . . .

• **Digestive enzymes without betaine hydrochloride.** These aid digestion and are often a problem in teens with skin problems of all sorts. Take immediately following meals, and get one with similar amounts to Super Enzyme™ by Twinlab™—but without betaine hydrochloride.

And, for the Postmenopausal Set, I Might Add . . .

• **Digestive enzymes with betaine hydrochloride.** Most people over forty need additional stomach acid to help with digestion, and it's added to good enzyme preparations. My recommendation is Super Enzyme™ by Twinlab™. You can take one after meals, and if there are no side effects, you can try two, but not more, and never before meals. Both skin and digestion problems tend to be helped at the same time. You might be pleasantly surprised with this, but digestion improvements tend to occur first. If meals clear more quickly and gas is decreased, then in time your skin may start healing more readily and hold moisture better.

• **Bioflavonoids.** For some reason, postmenopausal women often have additional problems with bruising, which is not improved with vitamin C alone. Adding 1,000 mg of bioflavonoids can be very beneficial in this area.

We obviously can barely scratch the surface of skin problems in these few pages. However, the rules for at least starting to deal with even more serious ones are outlined here, since any problems with the body require the integrated teamwork of the basic nutrients before adding others for specific problems.

CHAPTER 18

Nutrition and Your Child's Behavior

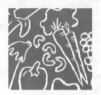

WHEN YOU CONSIDER your child's behavior, do you see anything "abnormal"? Is the attention span measured in microseconds? Is there unreasonable irritability or anger, or is there even what you'd consider bizarre behavior? How about a "slow thinker"? Does the kid have one of those neat labels, like "learning disability," "attention deficit disorder," or "hyperactivity"? Or worse, is your child's behavior driving you crazy, while the "experts" are telling you it's normal? I have seen kids systematically destroy my office in minutes, while the parents are told the behavior is normal or even that they are to blame for being poor disciplinarians. Of course, if it's bad enough that the teacher can't handle it or the doctor wants to kill the monster, then we're told that drugs are the answer.

The real question is, if these behaviors are observed, is there anything you can actually do about it without resorting to a prescription? The answer, over 90 percent of the time, is a resounding, nontoxic yes.

Bear in mind, we're trying to discuss most childhood behaviors in just a few pages (Dr. Spock would go crazy). Given the multitude of causes of altered behavior in children, the undertaking might seem a fairly ludicrous idea, I guess, except that biochemi-

cally oriented therapists have been treating these situations for
years with truly remarkable results. Once you entertain the idea
that behavior may have a biochemical basis, tracking down the
cause can be exciting, and it quite possibly might not be all that
difficult. Even those who feel the cause to be environmental (i.e.,
strictly emotional) often find behavior to be biochemically aggra-
vated, if not actually biochemically caused.

Areas to consider in this approach include the following:

• Food Allergy/Chemical Sensitivity
• Yeast
• Malnourishment (intake and/or absorption)
• Biochemical Imbalances

One simplifying factor to this technique, in my opinion, is that
the behavior label often is not that significant. How the child man-
ifests the biochemical problem is less important than the fact that
there is one. Track it down, handle it, and be done with it.
(Actually, you may have to control it, so you can't totally be done
with it, but the absence of the undesirable behavior makes the
effort amazingly worthwhile.)

Food Allergy and Chemical Sensitivity

This is the simplest, largest, and most rewarding area within
which to start your hunt for a biochemical behavior solution. Right
off the bat, you must remove nonfood chemicals from the child's
diet. This is no joke, and the potential rewards of this simple step
are well worth the effort. All artificial flavors, colors, preservatives
(other than vitamin C), and enhancers (MSG, etc.), need to be
removed for at least one week (one lifetime would be better).

If the child's behavior, whatever it is, is worse in the first three
to four days, you almost absolutely are on the right track.
Assuming things are better after a week, you can track down
offending agents by reintroducing them, one at a time, and observ-
ing the results. This trick alone may make a believer out of you.

There are two specific chemical groups of which to be particularly suspicious. One is the salicylate group, which, besides aspirin, exists naturally in most fruits and also in green peppers, chili peppers, vinegar, cucumbers, pickles, and other foods. The other is caffeine, which of course is in soft drinks, coffee, tea, chocolate, and some pain medications. (Excellent authors for further study in this area include Ben Feingold, M.D., and Doris Rapp, M.D.)

Next, look for actual foods that may have adverse effects. These can be items you have always considered excellent foods, and they most likely will be ones you use every day. Any food the child craves, or eats every day, must be eliminated for one week. The hardest to stop is usually sugar, a major offender. (The question of whether refined sugar is actually a food at all is discussed more at length in Chapter 2.)

Again, if behavior deteriorates in the first few days, stick it out; you are onto something. In fact, if the child misses the food so badly that your actual existence is threatened, you are almost guaranteed an improved child at the end of the test period. You can challenge the kid with the food later to see if you can turn on and off the offending behavior. At this point you may actually get the child on your side. Nobody wants to feel bad.

A small piece of sexist bad news is that the men in the family tend to be poorer observers of altered behavior. A representative tale is that of the mother coming home and finding her child merrily peeling tiles off the ceiling with his teeth. She accuses the father of having given an offending agent, to which he replies, "How could you tell? I only gave him one!"

For the mothers, do any of you recall, during your pregnancy, the experience of carrying a hyperactive gymnast type who was constantly kicking you to pieces? If so, could you make any association with what you had just eaten? This is a good early way to look for sensitivities, even before birth.

Beware, here's a biggie: the worst potential troublemaker for your child, both behaviorally and physically, is cow's milk. If there are behavior changes after coming off the breast, allied with recurrent ear problems, please test the child for dairy allergy. This test may take up to twenty-one days to ensure accurate results. (Dairy

186 · Nutritionally Incorrect

sensitivity may show a delayed response, so the standard seven-day evaluation period can be inadequate.).

Be patient, and be absolutely certain milk is not a problem before releasing the child to have it ad lib. This can (but may not) include cheese, cream, and butter, too, so be careful. Cow's milk is for baby cows, and once it's pasteurized and homogenized it isn't even fit for them! (For the record, the answer to the common question of calcium in the diet is that children get calcium the same way that cows get it: green, leafy plants, or, for breast feeders, from mothers who eat similar plants.)

After milk, the top five offending foods are wheat, corn, eggs, citrus, and sugar. Statistically, wheat is number two, and it's in everything, so this may take a bit of effort to test. It is often worth it, so try to last the week. (For further reading, try Lendon Smith, M.D., Ben Feingold, M.D., or William Crook, M.D.)

Yeast

This may be an allergy problem in older kids who have been fighting years of infections, usually middle ear and others, such that many courses of antibiotics have been given. Cortisone, prednisone, and other medications can contribute, so prolonged histories of taking these drugs should also be suspect. Intestinal problems, particularly diarrhea, indicate a disruption of the normal state of bacterial flora in the body, which allows for an invasion by common yeasts, which are everywhere in nature, but kept at a reasonable level in the body by normally adequate immune defenses.

A stressed immune system, however, can permit overgrowth of these organisms, with worsening abdominal complaints, and gradually manifesting behavior problems, such as listlessness, difficulty concentrating, apathy, and irritability. Thrush, a yeast infection in the mouth, and diaper rash (or jock itch for the older kids), along with red, moist rashes in skin fold areas, and athlete's foot should cause a high degree of suspicion.

Treatment consists of several efforts:

• Enhancing the immune system by using nutritional supplementation so that antibiotics are needed less frequently;
• Reestablishing the normal bacterial state in the gastrointestinal tract;
• Avoiding yeast-containing foods;
• Utilizing agents that kill yeast systemically.

The key to normal flora in the gut is the use of a beneficial bacteria called *Lactobacillus acidophilus* (*L. acidophilus*). Though commonly dairy based, health food stores carry both dairy and nondairy types. Usually the latter type comes in powder or capsule form, given before meals and at bedtime. If abdominal complaints decrease, usually behavior follows with an improvement.

Besides treating the gut, high-yeast foods should be avoided, at least for awhile. These include breads, starches, mushrooms, and anything fermented or leavened (this means the mother must not eat these foods, if she is breast-feeding). Yeasts feed on simple carbohydrates, so the sugars need to be avoided at first, then individually tested. Candy, cake, etc., of course are totally out, but this list can also include fruits, which at least should be left out for the first week. Melons, strawberries, and fresher, less sweet fruits should be reintroduced first.

If efforts in this area start to show results, then antiyeast agents may be necessary to finish the job. Over-the-counter (health-food store) preparations include caprylic acid and tannic acid, herbal tea (taheebo or pau d'arco), and other combination agents. My favorite, however, is olive leaf extract, followed by grapefruit (not grape, in this case) seed extract.

It's even possible that more will be necessary to fully alleviate the situation, which could require the intervention of a nutritionally oriented physician. These practitioners may use antiyeast medications, with names such as nystatin, Diflucan™, Sporanox™, and/or Nizoral™. Further reading here should definitely include William Crook, M.D., Orian Truss, M.D., Luc de Schepper, M.D., or John Trowbridge, M.D., all having written books on this underdiagnosed and underappreciated illness caused by our "civilized" fad diet and chemicalized "civilized" living. See the Appendix for more information.

Malnourishment

In our modern civilization, what people think of as "malnutrition" is admittedly rare. However, most people think that as long as calories and protein are adequate, there is no problem with poor nourishment. Talk about nothing being farther from the truth!

Our foods are awash in "naked" calories, meaning that what used to be good food is now processed and refined to the point that the nutrients required for the assimilation of the food have been removed from it. The point is that enough is removed, including fiber, that the food is concentrated and no longer in its natural state, which lends it more readily to the generation of sensitivities.

Most important, since the nutrients required for the food's absorption are gone, those nutrients will be taken from the body's own stores, which is why nutritional deficiencies are caused. This is why a food is not a food unless it's "complete," otherwise it becomes a stress on the body, which must use its own stores to handle the item's breakdown into usable parts. (There's that nutrient density issue again.)

As most of our foods are refined, including cereals, breads, pastas, grains, desserts, sugars, etc., nutritional deficiencies abound, in my opinion, and changes in behavior soon follow. This is a major reason to obtain really whole foods as much as possible.

Once fiber is removed, starches break down to sugar faster, and sugars get into the system even faster still, causing too rapid increases in blood sugar, with corresponding insulin overcorrections by the pancreas to bring the blood sugar back down. This is reactive hypoglycemia, and talk about behavior changes! Temper outbursts, irritability, lethargy (depending upon where in the cycle the person is), confusion, fatigue, apathy are all possibilities. If you cannot concentrate, you cannot learn; if you cannot learn, then you are "learning disabled," and you've earned a new label!

So, get the kids off refined foods. Make the rice brown rice, the barley dehulled only, the wheat 100 percent stone ground, the pasta whole grain, and trash the refined sugar. The kids will rebel, go nuts, and then they'll feel better, after which maybe you can reason with them.

Besides bad food, low blood sugar, and stressed nutrient stores, another problem is that many kids do not absorb even good foods very well, due to poor enzyme systems, poor beneficial bacteria, poor vitamin levels, poor eating habits (your kid does eat slowly and chew thoroughly, right?), or other causes. This is another factor that allows even lower nutrient levels in the body, both vitamins and minerals, and some of them are definitively linked to changes in behavior.

I am solidly of the opinion that we all need supplemental doses of nutrients; the Recommended Daily Allowances are inadequate, and our foods rarely even supply those meager amounts.

The best-known nutrients associated with behavior are vitamins C, B6, pantothenic acid (B5), niacin/niacinamide (B3), and the minerals chromium, zinc, manganese and magnesium. All of these might be given to a child with learning or behavioral problems. It is easier to underdose than to give too much (I believe kids are underdosed all the time), and with few exceptions, the body removes what it does not want.

Vitamins act as a team, however, and at least the B-complex should be taken all together before selecting individual nutrients for specialized purposes. This is true not only for behavior, but also for any health problem using a nutritionally oriented approach.

Biochemical Imbalances

Unfortunately, it's possible for all sorts of genetic defects to cause biochemical weaknesses in the functioning of the body. There are rare ones, like the XYY Syndrome in males, which is known for excessively violent behavior.

However, it's the occurrence of less specific abnormalities that can cause problems, about many of which it is possible to do something. We have already mentioned hypoglycemia, with its wide swings in blood sugar levels. This can be due to the use of inappropriate foods, or a person can be genetically predisposed to such swings, even without a particularly disgraceful diet.

If your child is a "Jekyll and Hyde" type, rapidly changing back and forth from angel to demon, and food sensitivities are not involved (I'll bet they are though), then consider hypoglycemia. Besides an unrefined diet, space the consumption of that diet into multiple small meals, or even allow nearly constant snacking. Try very hard to slow the time it takes to eat, and have the child chew thoroughly whatever is eaten. In this way, the next blood sugar rise helps offset the previous blood sugar low.

Hypoglycemia is a stress on the pancreas, and supplementation with chromium, in the form of GTF (glucose tolerance factor) chromium or chromium picolinate, can be noticeably helpful. Low-dose vanadium, in the form of vanadyl sulfate, may also be beneficial. Often these children are low in manganese, also, from constant ingestion of refined sugar. If there are real doubts as to the diagnosis, a five-hour glucose tolerance test can be very revealing. (Less than five hours is not enough.)

Technically, reactive hypoglycemia, or an over response to sugar challenge, is considered more of a symptom than a disease. It tells you to keep looking for a cause.

Pyroluria causes the urine to have detectable levels of something called the mauve factor. This causes a combined deficiency of both zinc and vitamin B6, and can cause antisocial behavior. (Carl Pfeiffer, M.D., Ph.D., and Abram Hoffer, M.D., Ph.D., both have books discussing this subject, but they are difficult to find.)

Histadelia has measurably high levels of histamine in the blood. This is more common in addictive types of behavior. Both of the above are dealt with at the the Carl Pfeiffer Treatment Center, Naperville, Illinois (Dr. Wm. Marsh).

A large area of consideration for altered behavior is that of tissue levels of metals, both high and low. Blood testing may pick up some of these, but the simplest and least expensive way is by hair analysis. High-tissue copper (water pipes, cookware, etc.), lead (paint, exhaust fumes, etc.), cadmium (cigarette smoke, air pollution, water pollution), aluminum (cookware, antiperspirants, soft

Labs Offering Hair Tests

Great Smokies Diagnostics, Asheville, NC
  800-522-4762; 828-253-0621; www.gsdl.com

Doctor's Data, Chicago, IL
  800-323-2784; 630-377-8139; www.doctorsdata.com

Omegatech, P.O. Box 1, Ripshin Rd., Troutdale, VA 24378
  800-437-1404; 440-835-2150;
  www.kingjamesomegatech-lab.com

drink cans), and mercury (water pollution, contaminated fish, etc.) can all cause your child to think like a slug, which opens one up to all sorts of nasty labels.

On the low side, chromium and manganese are often victims of high-sugar diets, being consumed to handle the refined sugars. Tissue zinc can also be a factor, especially when abnormal behavior is accompanied by skin problems (see Chapter 17).

Hair testing is inexpensive and easy, though not always reliable. The problem is finding a doctor who will order it. All naturopaths will, and most chiropractors will also. Your doctor may need a little coaxing, but give it a shot.

Behavior problems will always be with us, as parents, guardians, teachers, coaches, tour guides, whatever. They will not disappear, but excesses in behavior need to be recognized for what they are—unnecessary excesses, often controllable by a little study, concern, and effort aimed at what fuel we pump into our kids and how it's done. Don't give up, and don't fall prey to accusations of poor parenting or poor discipline. (Unless it's true!)

Keep reading. See the Appendix for book lists for all the subject areas we discuss, and pick away at the areas that interest you most.

Best of luck in your quest for the perfect child. Such a thing may not exist, but your efforts toward that end may be richly rewarded nonetheless. The answer *is* out there—somewhere.

For the Older and Wiser

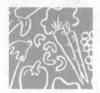

AH, THE "GOLDEN AGE." The elderly. Those revered by society as "sages," the "holders of wisdom," the "keepers of knowledge," enlightened and perceptive giants we treat with awe and respect, hanging on their every word.

When's the last time you thought of our senior citizens in such a manner? Has our advancement in technology just passed them by? Has our faster pace left them behind? Something happened, because in most of the civilizations of the past, the elderly were respected in just such a way. Now they're just old.

All of us need to be very careful. Short of accidents, wars, or "the Big One, Ethel," we're all going to get there—old, that is. Some of us sooner than others, and I don't mean by reaching age 65. Haven't you seen people who look 55 and then you find out they're 68? Or someone whose age you happen to know is 41, but looks 55?

What's going on here? Just a case of good genes/bad genes? God's will? Karma? What about senility, Alzheimer's disease, arthritis, osteoporosis, diabetes, incontinence, helplessness, hopelessness? Just a question of fate? If that's so, why have all the above "common problems" of the elderly only hit us in the last 50 to 100 years? We've been around quite a bit longer than that.

The point is most of the curses afflicting the elderly today are not only fairly new but they are occurring earlier and earlier—descending well into middle age. And they aren't just from poverty. There are some awfully wealthy arthritic Alzheimer's patients around.

I believe there are real things we can do about many of them. To put things into proper perspective, the health problems of the elderly are an outgrowth of decades of stresses: poor food quality, poor digestion, and subsequent lousy absorption; decreasing exercise, often from feeling too bad to pursue it; toxins of all types in our air, water, and food; tons of prescription medications; and of course bad genes are in there, too.

Obviously we're not going to erase them all. The problems didn't get that way overnight, and we can't bypass every genetic or biochemical tendency inherent in each individual. However, there are several specific stresses we can do something about that affect almost all the elderly across the board. By working on those, sometimes the difference is nothing short of amazing.

Anyway, getting started obviously involves initiating the basic plan (Chapter 20). The good news here is that it is not necessary to worry about whether the diet is "balanced." That is a much-overrated phrase, and for senior citizens living alone it can be enough to put the person off trying a new diet right from the start.

As long as the general dietary rules are followed, there is often change for the better noticed within two to four weeks, even without starting vitamins (which definitely should be done). You can imagine that it tends to take a bit longer than with younger adults, and longer still than with children. The longer it took to get in the fix you're in, the longer to crawl back out!

Some people can do without digestive enzymes, but very rarely are the elderly in that category. My experience has been that I've yet to find a "senior" who didn't benefit from them. Apparently after all those years the enzyme batteries just need a little extra charging to help them along. However, not all require (or can take) the betaine hydrochloride that is contained in many brands. I would start with one that has it, as most need it, then fall back to one without it if there is any indigestion or burning.

There are tests for the status of the stomach environment, but they can be hard to locate; and the trial-and-error approach, if done cautiously, is adequate and cheaper.

A last note on the diet. Many senior citizens can't chew. They may have the time to enjoy a meal and eat it slowly; they just don't have good dentition anymore. Food processors and pureeing foods to make them "pre-chewed" can be invaluable. Another highly nutritious solution can be the easily digestible cell foods, like spirulina, chlorella, barley green, and/or blue-green algae—magnificent additions to the diet of the denture wearer (or anyone).

A really major way for the elderly to cruise past a signpost of progress on our health highway is to make absolutely certain that every single prescription they are taking is absolutely necessary. If it isn't absolutely necessary, then absolutely get off it. (Check with your doctor to see if it must be tapered first . . . it's amazing how dangerous some of these drugs are.)

I have seen people in an almost zombie state from long lists of medications; we all have, I bet. Doctors are busy people and are trained to treat a symptom with a drug, sometimes without being aware that the patient is experiencing a symptom from a drug obtained from another doctor. When I was monitoring a home for the elderly, it was a general occurrence to see ten drugs on a medication list. I remember one with eighteen!

Sometimes just getting off the drugs can deliver a new human being. With good food, the time to eat it correctly, and well-absorbed nutritional supplements, it's not at all uncommon for family members to notice a new alertness and energy in individuals formerly written off as senile and weak.

What's worse, new prescription drugs are emerging in the market all the time. In fact, it's happening faster now than ever before. So fast, in fact, that it's clear to me that they cannot possibly all be tested long term. That means the chronic (long-term) effects of such medications are totally unknown, and most likely due to make themselves known in the population of our elderly. Only if the side effects are so bad that they just don't stay on the market do the seniors have a chance (and that frequently does happen).

Before any new drug is added to a senior's medication list, make sure of two rules:

1. It is absolutely necessary.
2. It has a previously established track record of tolerable long-term side effects. Remember that such a record is rare.

There's one other thing about drug therapies: There are well-established nutritional therapies for a huge number of signs and symptoms. These types of possibilities should at least be considered before a senior takes, or is encouraged to take, prescription drugs. One of the best sources is *Prescription For Nutritional Healing*. See the Appendix for this and other literature suggestions.

A last comment on drugs: just because a medication is not prescription (i.e., over-the-counter) does not mean that drug is harmless. For one thing, more and more prescription drugs are becoming available over the counter because there is such a huge market for them. They aren't any less toxic when the prescription label is removed. In fact, if anything at all is done, it is usually to take the original drug and provide it in half-strength doses. Take two and you have the original prescription dose. Hardly much difference.

What's worse is that our elderly, like the rest of us, have been brainwashed into the fixation that over-the-counter drugs are so weak or so safe, that they can be ingested by the pound without difficulties. I have known elite athletes (gymnasts and divers), from age ten to take over-the-counter pain killers by the handfuls. A few helped, at first, then the pain got worse, so they increased the dose until they got some kind of relief. No relief, increase the dose . . . they're harmless of course, so no prolem. Imagine pursuing that concept for sixty or seventy years.

Few of us drink enough water. The elderly are famous for this mistake. We're not talking coffee, tea, and soft drinks here; we're talking water. Abram Hoffer, M.D., Ph.D., a long-time expert in the use of high-dose nutrients in the treatment of both mental and other illnesses believes many of those who are senile are chronically dehydrated. Several months of good water, eight glasses a day, may offer significant improvement. When added to good food and supplements, you may knock down those signposts on the road to senior citizenship by the stack!

If there's one thing that the elderly have had time to do, it's to get toxic. Whatever the nasty bug sprays, fertilizers, weed killers, hormones, industrial wastes and vehicle exhausts we've all been consuming, seniors have been doing it longer. And, like the commercial said about their spaghetti sauce, "It's in there."

They're in there, all right, and the effects add up. Drinking reasonable amounts of good water is a great help, but after such a long time spent exposed to so many chemical insults, it usually isn't enough.

Detoxifying is a huge subject of its own, but if the senior is willing to make changes and swallow some supplements anyway, a great simple detoxifier is good ol' vitamin C (see Chapter 9). High doses (grams, not milligrams) are magnificent aids to helping the body's liver, kidneys and fatty storage depots handle years of built-up chemical stresses.

For seniors, it may be simpler to start with ascorbate forms of vitamin C instead of ascorbic acid. These are nonacidic, and calcium, magnesium and other minerals can also be given at the same time, depending upon the type used. When swallowed as capsules or taken mixed in food as a powder, they are usually well absorbed. (V8 Juice and tomato juice are good vehicles for this, as they hide undesirable tastes well—vitamin C is either sour or bitter.)

Of all the chemical stresses, I'm going to pick one as the worst for the elderly. In my opinion, the most widespread danger, at least to mental health, is aluminum. Not because it's an acute killer, like arsenic, but because it's absolutely everywhere. In the elderly, with decades to build up a body-wide supply, there's no telling how badly they're being affected.

What's worse is the big brothers at FDA don't even recognize the stuff as that bad. Unlike lead, cadmium and nickel, known to be toxic, aluminum only sits in a suspicious sort of category. They have said, however, that fifty parts per million (ppm) in a soda can should be tolerable. What they haven't bothered to tell us is that an aluminum soda can, after three months, may have up to 6,000 ppm, and available evidence shows measurably higher absorption in humans from drink-can use! (Acres, U.S.A. 1994; Gerrans 1992). No one has any idea of such effects. We haven't had aluminum cans long enough. That's why tin cans hung around so long; tin doesn't leach into the contents. Unfortunately, the big aluminum interests had their way.

Most people have heard that there is a link between aluminum buildup and Alzheimer's disease. If there ever were a new-age disease for our elderly, this is it. It's a recent syndrome known only to our modern civilization. If you ever have a loved one with this disease, you'll understand devastation.

So our senior citizen isn't into soft drinks? What about antiperspirants? Baking powder? Buffered aspirin? (Gee, I don't know any seniors who take that.) Antacids? (Or those.) Toothpaste? Many cosmetics? Food wrappers? Processed cheese? (Gaby 1997). These items can all be loaded with many milligrams of aluminum.

Obviously, it would be nice to avoid those sources as much as possible. If the senior already appears a bit senile, I would recommend a hair test, just like we did for the kids, which finds the levels of minerals deposited in hair and that includes aluminum. (See the Appendix for sources.) Should the level be high, one nontoxic remedy worth trying is homeopathic Ipecac, 6x potency, available at good health stores.

There's a lot more to the story of senility. A great place to learn more about its treatment is *Smart Nutrients—A Guide to Nutrients that Can Prevent and Reverse Senility* by Hoffer and Walker.

Of the chronic degenerative diseases associated with aging, the most disfiguring, painful, and notorious has to be arthritis. This is what turns a lively upright grandmother into a pretzel, up to a foot shorter than she used to be due to changes in the spine. It can completely ruin hand function, hip function, or almost any other joint function it pleases. You may have noticed the typical finger-to-hand joints that cause the victim's fingers to angle downward, away from the thumb. Eventually they can become nothing more than useless appendages. Ask anyone with the problem about the pain.

There absolutely are things you can do for this, especially if you start early enough before there is much joint destruction. The latest book on the subject and the one to make the most noise is *The Arthritis Cure* by Jason Theodosakis, M.D. However, he isn't the first to have something to contribute, nutritionally, to this horrible illness. Older, but excellent nonetheless, is the book *There Is a Cure for Arthritis,* by Paavo Airola, N.D.

As much of a nutrition nut as I am, I'm afraid I have to agree, at least to some extent, that exercise is important. You need to stimulate the circulatory system for adequate distribution of nutrients for one thing, though there are certainly far more benefits to exercise than that.

So how does an elderly person, maybe with a fair amount of arthritis, get any reasonable amount of exercise? The simplest way, of course, is to walk. You can do that anywhere, though maybe not in any weather. Jogging isn't necessary, and even getting out of breath isn't, though a little rise in pulse wouldn't hurt. Starting to walk, then gradually increasing the distance while staying in a comfortable state of exertion is wonderful, and most people feel better afterward.

If there is something the person considers truly fun, then the problem is solved. Just try to do a bit more of it, be it shuffleboard, bowling, horseshoes, rowing, whatever.

There is another way that is more convenient than walking and even better for you, if you really find that nothing strikes your fancy for fun exercise. It doesn't require going out; you can do it during your favorite TV show, and you don't even have to get dressed. It's magnificent for the circulation, even if you don't do enough to get tired. It's easier on the joints than walking, and it's really fun. It's a trampoline. Yeah, picture that—Granny somersaulting on a trampoline.

Actually, the trampoline we're talking about is the small circular one called a mini tramp. The utility of these things is truly incredible and, if you shop around, the price is right. An exciting thing about these devices is that they offer benefits without doing anything more than just moving up and down on the balls of the feet. That's why seniors can get so much out of them, even if they are arthritic. It isn't necessary to actually bounce on either one foot or two. Merely by rocking up and down there is a large increase in the movement of blood from the lower extremities and to the rest of the body, even if the person has poor valves in the veins of the legs. The balls of the feet never need to leave the surface of the tramp.

So, be it rain or shine, hot or cold, dressed or undressed, you can bounce (or just rock) during your favorite TV show. It's hard to cook up an excuse—other than you just plain refuse—and it really is easy enough and fun enough that developing the habit isn't hard at all. For the bounce-and-watch-TV types, like me, I recommend one with bungee cords instead of metal springs; they don't squeak.

There are even mini-tramps with railings on both sides for those who need them. I've seen it done with an elderly gentleman using a cane in each hand, and very lightly pursuing the up and down motion. If the person is truly infirm, I don't know that I can recommend it for safety reasons, but you will have to use your own judgment on this one. (Actually, you'll have to use your own judgment on all of 'em, whatever you're doing.)

Finally, there is no substitute for working out the brain. Like any other organ—use it or lose it—so be sure to stimulate the intellect. Short of full-blown senility or Alzheimer's disease, there should be something that can be used to stimulate everyone's concentration. If you're not the reading type, check out something else. From solitaire to crossword puzzles, there are all levels of difficulty. Jigsaw puzzles, riddles, picture puzzles, manual puzzles (like Rubik's Cube, etc.) all offer a stimulus to concentrate, and it helps to have the brain work on stuff like that.

There must be something every senior can enjoy applying the brain cells to. If it can be done with others, that's the best way. It offers not only interaction but also incentive, if a group is involved.

Find it. Do it. Your grandchildren will thank you.

The Plan

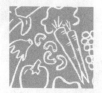

CHAPTER 20

The Plan

THIS IS IT. Whether you've read all the preceding drivel isn't really important if I can get you to try the plan anyway. However, the odds are better if you understand why one would want or need to do all the things listed. Many may make sense right off, but some might need other chapters in order to provide a rationale for the beginner.

However you try it, just try it. Please. A moderate effort for one month would be great because I can almost guarantee that you will feel better. Just one week might do it, but that's a bit of a gamble if you have lots of toxins or allergies aboard that you need to counteract.

Unfortunately, I don't have any financial interest in any of the suppliers suggested. They are purely examples that are prominent enough for beginners to find and use as a starting point. I sell only information, and now you have that, so my bias toward what I hope you will do is solely an outgrowth of research and clinical observations.

Dietary Guidelines

This is the basic diet for a starting point to optimum health. It is not a weight routine diet per se. Normally, an underweight person will gain some weight on this routine, while an overweight person will lose, following the same rules. This is not magic: the same rules can cause the poor absorber to absorb better, and the poor utilizer to better burn foods that were absorbed.

The Bad News

- No refined sugar—none, zero, zilch. (This is the goal, anyway.)
- No refined flour—Hang on, though, there's hope.
- Absolutely minimize milk—useless AT BEST (unless certified raw), even for calcium, low-fat or otherwise.
- Avoid chlorinated water (and any city water) for drinking. Evian® is best if you can afford it, but there are also decent domestic brands if you try to find deep well sources. Be sure filters remove chlorine and fluoride.
- Minimize fruit juices, and dilute with water, if possible.
- Avoid caffeine, alcohol, and nicotine (what a drag—sorry!).
- Easy on red meats (two to three times per week, or get organic).
- Avoid mixing proteins (meat, eggs, cheese, nuts, seeds) with sugars, fruit, or starches at the same meal. (This is impossible to do 100 percent. However, the attempt aids digestion, as protein requires a higher-acid environment than the sugars, etc. In a similar way agents like antacids help ruin digestive efficiency.)
- No frying (or deep frying) of anything. (Wok-type or stir frying is okay.)
- Easy on artificial sweeteners. (Besides being toxic, they can be appetite stimulants.) Beware aspartame's side effects.
- Avoid processed foods (e.g., get natural peanut butter, cold-pressed, unprocessed oils, butter instead of margarine or "plastic butter;" say no to luncheon meats, smoked foods, hydrogenation, homogenization).
- Avoid additives (colorings, flavorings, MSG, preservatives, etc.). Read labels carefully!

- Beware of craved foods. (These could be anything.) Give each up for a week, then retry, looking for symptoms.
- Stop using aluminum cans. It leeches into the contents quickly.
- Eat slowly and chew thoroughly!
- Eat slowly and chew thoroughly!
- No kidding about the previous two bullets.

The Good News

- All the fresh fruits you want. Try to get unsprayed fruit so you can eat the skins. Entire fruit meals are fine. (Avoid grapes, dates and figs if you gain weight easily.)
- Eat a lot of veggies and legumes—raw, steamed, or wok fried. A little soy sauce is okay—experiment with spices instead of salt, if you retain fluid easily. (Snacking is okay.)
- Drink good water or herb teas as much as you want. Sweeten teas with fruit juice (as little as possible) or the herb stevia.
- Eat fish and fowl, either baked or broiled.
- Organ meats are okay—any way you can get 'em down. (Once a week for calf's liver if you have very high cholesterol). Avoid adult beef liver.
- For snacks, eat fresh (raw) nuts and seeds (natural nut butters, too). These are great appetite killers.
- Eggs are fine, free-range fertile are much better. Don't break the yolk in cooking. (Air and heat, together, change cholesterol into a bad form, when it's otherwise okay.)
- Cheese is okay in moderation; raw milk type is much better. Consider soy cheeses and tofu (both soft and firm types) for twenty-one days if dairy is not tolerated, to see if cheese is an exception.
- Butter is superior (by far!) to margarine, if you are not sensitive to it. Use the low salt types, which may also have less yellow dye in them. Whipped types allow you to use less, while thinking you are getting the same amount. Land 'o Lakes™ has some good ones. If you are butter sensitive, consider Spectrum Spread® by Spectrum Naturals®.
- Breads and grains are ideal if 100 percent whole (brown rice, whole wheat, dehulled barley, millet, oats, amaranth, etc.)

- Pasta is fine, all forms, as long as it's spinach type, artichoke type, 100 percent whole wheat, or brown rice type. It's heavy, so try angel hair and don't serve as much. You won't need as much.
- Use whole-grain cereals without sugar (fruit juice sweetened is okay). They're harder to find, but try health food stores.
- Unprocessed, raw flaxseed is the best oil you can get. (It has a slightly nutty flavor.) Also use virgin olive oil. Cold-pressed saf-flower oil is are acceptable if the others are unavailable. Avoid canola oil—it's a modified rape seed product and I don't trust it.
- For sweet cravings, try unsweetened applesauce, a little raw honey, or maybe a frozen banana. (Be creative—cinnamon toast, for example, is great, using raw honey and whole-grain bread.)
- Rice milk, almond milk, oat milk and soy milk are available to replace the cow somewhat. There are also flavored ones, besides just plain. (Children should avoid soy due to estrogen-like com-pounds.)
- If you slip up and junk out, don't quit! You might even need an occasional "Junk Day." Just do it, write it off, and get back on track. (Check out fruit juice-sweetened bars and cookies at health food stores, and nowadays, even at better supermarkets.)

Such a routine is not meant to be torture. It's the way mankind was meant to eat. If diligently tried, most people find many of their tastes begin to change, causing natural foods to become far more palatable. Again, a "junk day" is preferable to not playing the game at all.

Note: If you try the plan and feel worse in the first few days, you are probably experiencing food-sensitivity withdrawal. This is typ-ically a good sign, as improvement starting by day four or five can have you feeling better than ever.

Survival Tips

- Easy does it where change is concerned. Trying to change every-thing at once may mean you won't stick with the plan. Make a few changes at first that seem the most reasonable to you, then a few more, and a few more. Gradually your taste buds will change and healthy food will taste better than junk.

- Kids love hot dogs and health food stores actually carry healthy ones with no additives. Shelton's is one brand I know of that comes frozen—my niece and nephew have grown up on them.

- Kids love popsicles, too! My sister even has the neighborhood junk food kids asking for seconds of her organic fruit juice popsicles. She puts full strength juice in plastic popsicle makers. (This is the only place her kids get full strength juice, and popsicles are a treat, not a standard food. Other times juices are served half water and half juice.)

- Many health food cereals are not bad; granolas are a good place to start as they are often sweeter than other cereals; so sweet, in fact, that after awhile they can be wet with water, which will leach the dehydrated fruit juice back out, sweetening the whole thing.

- Ask around to find a health food co-op where you can buy healthy foods wholesale. Besides saving money, the members can tell you which foods are worth trying and which just taste like cardboard.

- Many newcomers to health foods actually like veggie burgers. I recommend those made mostly from grains rather than soy to start. Serve on whole-wheat rolls like hamburgers or with a sauce like salisbury steak. This one may be a hit, and with the whole-wheat buns, they are really filling.

- Use your public library for cookbooks and ideas. Copy the recipes you like and return the book! Some of the Seventh Day Adventist cookbooks are said to have good vegetarian recipes.

- A rice cooker/steamer can make preparing healthy meals much easier and they are not that expensive.

- There are healthy chips and snacks that taste okay, but popcorn is probably one of the least expensive healthy snacks (assuming, of course, that you aren't allergic to it like I am . . . what a craving!).

- Oatmeal is both a good tasting and filling breakfast. You can even microwave it while you're getting dressed: two cups water to one cup oats in a covered casserole for fourteen minutes at 50 percent power, then add honey and vanilla or two mashed ripe bananas. You can also experiment with other grains cooked overnight in the crockpot to greet you in the morning.

• Whole-wheat or multigrain pancakes actually taste better than white. Try fruit juice as a syrup or use real maple syrup (easy now on this one as it's very concentrated), raw honey (remember that the bee does some refining of her own), apple butter, nut butters, rice syrup or just butter for a nice weekend breakfast. Make the pancakes in the shape of Mickey Mouse's head or the first letter of a child's name for kudos.

• I know this is heresy, but I am not against salt. However, it has to be really good salt, almost impossible to find in the U.S., and expensive. "Sea salt" is a deception in almost all cases. It's from the sea, but the minerals have been removed, which is why you wanted it in the first place. There are two companies that make a real salt that maintains its original mineral content. See the Appendix for their contact information.

Supplement Guidelines

Have a local medical professional monitor your status, should you decide to use any of this information. (There can be reactions to anything, so your own physician could be useful here. Someone with previous experience in nutrition therapies, of course, would be the best.)

The introduction of supplements for the first time should commence with one new nutrient every couple of days, so that, if any reaction should occur, you have a good idea how to track it down.

Avoid hard pills (go with capsules and powders, if possible), and avoid the use of timed-release types. They are more expensive, and you are paying extra for a pill that is deliberately designed not to break down immediately. Do your own time releasing, by when and how often you take something.

• **A *good multivitamin/mineral*:** Consider NOW Vit-Min 75+ Iron Free™, Solgar Multi-Nutrient™, Solaray Multi-Energy™ or Twinlab Daily Two Caps™ for a start. Most come with or without iron. (There are many others that are comparable.) These come with or without iron. Yours should be without iron and should stay that way unless your serum ferritin blood test falls below fifteen or your doctor says to take it. (Really good vitamin companies offer multivitamins minus iron, due to recent research showing that iron supplements can cause side effects and other problems.)

The recommended dose is one capsule twice a day. (Solaray, for example, has a three times a day dose that is stronger. If you wish, you might switch to this after the first bottle of another.)

There are other excellent brands, but these are readily available. Avoid the types that only have 100 percent of the U.S. Recommended Dietary Allowances (RDA). These lower nutrient brands are more expensive for what they contain, and the strengths are too low in my opinion. Plus they are all hard tablets. Compare labels, and buy accordingly. One hard tablet that really isn't bad, in price, dissolvability, and strength, is the multi from Health Watchers System, 800-321-6917, 631-567-9500, www.puritan.com.

Note: The ultimate multivitamin supplement is called Life Extension Mix™, but it costs more, of course, and involves taking up to fourteen capsules per day. This is usually reserved for the serious vitamin enthusiast. For excellent nutrition information you should call the Life Extension Foundation, 800-841-5433, 954-766-8433, www.lef.org.

Note: If you enjoy the multilevel, or network marketing, type of distribution, one choice would be Body Wise International. Their multivitamins are called Right Choice A.M. and Right Choice P.M. formulas. You can contact them for a distributor in your area at 800-239-9735 or www.bodywise.org.

Be careful using this method of attaining vitamins, especially if you wish to try my type of fairly high-dose plan. There are some well-made products that have doses too low for substantial effect, in my opinion.

- *Vitamin C:* You might start with 1,000 mg capsules at a daily dose of one capsule twice a day. If that is tolerated without stomach distress, consider increasing the dose to one capsule, three times a day. (If there is any stomach problem, you might try the ascorbate form, or the type called ester C. These are usually well tolerated, but cost a bit more.)

- **Digestive Enzymes:** Many adults do not make enough of these highly beneficial aids to the absorption process, so it might be worth a trial of augmenting by supplementation. The brand with which I usually start is Super Enzyme™ by Twinlab, at one capsule immediately after meals. If this is tolerated without any gastric distress, you might increase to two capsules after meals, but not more than two—and not before meals. You want to enhance what your body has made, not take its place.

   If there are gastric difficulties with this product, you can try one (there are many to choose from) that does not contain betaine hydrochloride. This is a stomach acid aid that is added to the enzymes in many products, since it is easy to be deficient in both.

   You want to make sure the enzymes are full spectrum (those which contain proteolytic, lipolytic, and amylolytic fractions). Your doctor can also supply these as a prescription item, under the name (there are others) of Pancrease MT-10™. I don't consider papaya or pineapple enzymes alone to be adequate.

- **Other/Miscellaneous:** Once you have been on the above supplement routine for about a month, only then consider additions tailored to meet your own personal situation. If at that point you think there is something to it, then it's time to play with specific problem areas that concern you directly. The best reference book for such a task is the following, available in health food stores and better bookstores: *Prescription For Nutritional Healing* by Balch & Balch. This isn't the kind of text you read cover to cover. You look up your problem, and see what it recommends. This is the best reference I've ever found for this purpose, but pills alone won't do it—you must know how to eat!

   If a good health food store is not nearby or if you want to price shop, here are a few nutritional supplement catalog companies you might try:

- VitaminUSA: (toll-free) 877-338-4826, 419-423-9875, fax: 419-423-1789, www.vitaminusa.com (A huge inventory and my favorite, cause they print my articles!)
- Willner Chemists: 800-633-1106, 212-682-2817, fax: 212-682-6192, www.willner.com
- The Vitamin Shoppe: 800-223-1216, 201-866-7711, www.vitaminshoppe.com
- Vitamin Wholesalers, Inc.: 800-848-6896, 954-563-0994, www.vitaminwholesalers.com
- Health Watchers System: 800-321-6917, 631-567-9500, www.puritan.com (These are hard pills, and large, but they break down well and the prices are reasonable.)
- Puritan's Pride: 800-645-1030, www.puritan.com (They have many hard pills, but some good prices; they're now combined with Health Watchers.)

Often there are cheaper prices available at local cooperatives, though they are harder to locate. Always compare. Remember that all catalog prices are not the same—even when they handle the same manufacturers!

Exercise

- If you exercise moderately at least three times per week, and enjoy it, keep it up.
- Find something you really like, if at all possible.
- If you don't exercise, or dislike what you do enough to consider quitting, get a mini trampoline with bungee-type springs.
- Start slow.
- Vary the type and intensity of bouncing.
- Bounce while watching TV shows, while listening to music, or other convenient periods. Try to keep going for at least a half-hour, but don't get too winded. Switch to keeping the balls of the feet on the tramp bed, only bouncing on your heels, if you're getting out of breath (toe wobbling).
- Work your way up slowly. Don't try to become a marathon run-

ner overnight! You'll either get into trouble, or you'll quit, neither of which does you any good.

- Try to do it (bounce, that is) at least three times per week.
- If you wish, you can consider getting aerobic, three times per week. Subtract your age from 220, then take 80 percent of that for your target pulse rate. Consider staying at that rate for twenty minutes. (Remember, check with your doc first.)
- "Wake up call" sit ups. Right when you wake up, before your eyes are even open, slide down in the bed (on your back) until your heels catch the mattress. Leave the covers on, and do some standard sit ups.
- Work your way up, slowly, and remain at a number you will continue to do, no matter how low it is, rather than getting too aggressive too early and quitting.

CHAPTER 21

Navigating Those Health Food Aisles

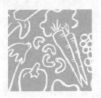

UNFORTUNATELY, THIS CHAPTER may not apply to every nation. In some countries drugs are easier to get than vitamins! Hopefully that's a trend that can be stopped. With the advent and expansion of the Internet, virtual health food stores are becoming more and more prominent, as our lists of web sites indicate. Maybe someday all food aisles will be "health food" aisles!

Basic Navigation Rules

If you've come this far you've covered a lot, in my opinion, especially if you really were a novice in nutrition and health. Now that you have the plan and know the basics of the supplements, it's time to add the details of their purchase and that of other "health foods," assuming that's the way you've decided to go.

It really can be pretty mind numbing: aisle upon aisle, row upon row, of endless quantities of intimidating bottles, each labeled with letters and numbers, or otherwise esoteric words that nobody can pronounce, much less understand. Is all of this just quackery? Is every customer of all these bottles just deluded—self-hyping on placebo effects and getting ripped off by some self-professed "expert" behind a checkout counter? Do these pills just cause expensive urine?

Questions like that are becoming easier to answer. Just by looking at the vast increase in the number of health food stores in the U.S., and the hugely expanding volume of patrons trying these "health-nut" ideas, it's apparent that something is going on, and they can't all be crazy. Now every drugstore and supermarket is following suit.

If you've read this far, or crossed the threshold of a health food store, or lingered at some supermarket's health food aisles, you at least probably have enough of an open mind to consider the possibility that there is something of real benefit going on here. The pills cost money, and the produce is always more expensive than a grocery chain, yet the demand as a whole (the subsequent number of stores) is growing.

Now, how does it all apply to you? Assuming you have the inclination, where do you begin? And what do you do to evaluate the potential of not only the mountains of bottles, but also the strange new variety of foods, drinks, snacks, cosmetics, devices, books and whatever else?

First of all, you must recognize that there are no absolutes about what's going on here. If your grandmother has finally browbeaten you into taking a few vitamins because they make her feel wonderful, there's no guarantee that the same ones will have the slightest effect on you. On the other hand, it's also possible that hers are not the only ones that have a history of successfully improving your symptoms.

Do any of them work? Is all this a giant placebo effect? (This is the very real observation that we may feel better merely because we are swallowing a pill to feel better. Since we're *supposed* to feel better, therefore we *do* feel better.) There certainly is something to the concept of mind over matter. If some of the effects of supplements take advantage of this, and you end up feeling better, who really cares? Keep your expensive urine (you're worth it) and continue to feel better!

Though by now I assume you've already decided to have an open mind on the subject; I feel obliged to comment that I have been using high doses of nutrient supplements for years, on myself, my family, my athletes, and my patients. I can state that supplements work, period. Whether they handle the specific problem you're having or whether they are the right dosage, well, that may be something else. It's certainly possible to improve your odds though, and the more you read (that is, the less of a beginner you are), the better your odds are of generating improvement.

Your "expensive urine" allows the body to pick and choose the types and quantities of nutrients it desires, as a rule. Everything is first thrown into the urine by the kidney, good and bad, with the good stuff reabsorbed farther along. If its absorptive capacity is poor, due to some suboptimal status of any of the thousands of enzymes in the body, less is returned to the body than would be by the so-called "average person."

The supplements, of course, are by far the biggest, and certainly the most intimidating, area of the store. But for the beginner, once you've learned to sail around those shelves full of every imaginable supplement with some degree of comfort, navigating the rest of the place isn't nearly so rocky. Besides, this is the good stuff.

Bear in mind, however, that this is a beginner's guide; there are entire books written on each nutrient, including some of the more esoteric ones we haven't even mentioned. If you find that some of the "rough waters" of your health status smooth out by using the basics, then you may wish to research further. (See Appendix.)

You need to keep two things in mind:

1. Supplements are not a replacement for food.
2. Supplements are usually taken with food.

Those All-Important Labels

• Absolutely mandatory is an understanding of the pill bottle label. Don't be intimidated, and don't ignore this part of your education. Read the labels, and by all means do it carefully!

- Don't worry about words you can't pronounce. Most of them are just chemical names, like tocopherol or pantothenate, that no one else understands either.
- Especially in multivitamins, but in other supplements also, companies precede their list of nutrients on the label with the words "two capsules provide," "six tablets provide," or something similar. Be sure you notice this, so you are comparing oranges to oranges when comparing prices. It's sneaky, in my opinion, but it's basically an accepted practice, so just look for it.
- Most pills are measured in milligrams (mg). There are 1,000 mg in 1 gram (g). This is the weight of the active ingredient being described. Some supplements are needed in such small doses that they are measured in micrograms (mcg). There are 1,000 mcg in just 1 mg (so the amount in these babies is small!).
- Fat-soluble vitamins are measured in international units (IU) because units of "activity" are more important than weight in these capsules. The same weight can have different activities, so this is a better way to compare strength in the fat solubles.
- Digestive enzymes are measured in gastric digestive units (GDU). This is a comparison of activity, so "GDU" is not a dirty word.
- Some supplements have cultures of active, "good guy" bacteria in them, like in yogurt. Their strength is measured in colony-forming units or (CFU).
- Ignore the size of the bottle. Instead, go with the number of pieces listed on the label. Let the buyer beware here. It's amazing what you may find.
- Some nutrients list a recommended daily allowance (RDA), established by something called a food and nutrition board. These will appear in a second column on the label and will be shown as a percentage of the RDA. Supplements having 100 percent of the RDA are normally a waste of time, as such a dose is merely to prevent overt deficiency syndromes from developing in someone called the "average person." As you probably aren't average and you want to do more than just prevent deficiencies, "the good stuff" will have considerably higher percentages than the RDA. Now, most are switching to " percent DV" (percent daily value), which is even lower.

- Following the list of goodies that are supposed to be in there, the manufacturer has to put on the label what else, if anything, is in the supplement that shouldn't be there. These include sugars, dyes, and inert ingredients (i.e., fillers, starch, and yeast, or the base in which everything's mixed, including its source). It's often worth knowing just what else you may be swallowing, especially if you are the allergic type.
- Finally, there will be a "directions" or "suggested dosage" line. Stay with this until you know more about what you're doing. It is not uncommon for well-informed users to exceed the label guidelines, but for the beginner, the saying "If a little is good, a lot is better" is not the way to go.

The "Multi" Shelves

We've covered the introduction to individual nutrients in Section 2, including the vitamins in Chapter 8. Having done that, I would say that very few newcomers to the habit of swallowing supplements should be picking from among too many of them. A lot of companies have dedicated themselves to doing that for you. This is where you pick your team, before concentrating on individual players. That keeps the starter plan in Chapter 20 easier.

It's possible someone told you that you just had to try a specific nutrient, and that's all you came in for. You ask the clerk, pay for it, and split. You don't even need to drop anchor. However, if you're in the market for educated good health, the multivitamin/minerals are the place to start. Here are some guidelines, many of which apply to most other supplements, as well.

- Capsules are almost always superior to hard pills. They are guaranteed to release quickly, so there is no worry that a person with poor digestion and/or absorption may not be breaking down a hard pill. (Then instead of expensive urine, you have expensive stool!) You also avoid sugar-coatings, unnecessary dyes, and the fillers that hold the pills together.

- If you must use hard pills, avoid time-release types, which are deliberately designed to not give you what's in them! The idea is to keep getting amounts of the supplement throughout the day, but many nutrients are only absorbed at certain points in the G.I. (gastrointestinal or digestive) tract; therefore amounts may be wasted.
- There's another reason to stay well above the RDA for the listed nutrients. In multivitamins it's easier to get more nutrient for the money. (Just compare labels with the common drug store brands.)
- Good multivitamins give you a choice on the label of with or without iron. Unless you are known to be anemic, proven through a blood test (serum ferritin), avoid the iron: it can constipate, and it readily causes free-radicals, real bad guys.
- Get as many minerals as possible included in the multiple. These make the pills bigger, but they save a lot of money and hassle and can be as important as the vitamins, if not more so.

So What Else Is There?

Foods and Snacks

Health food is better for you than regular food. A firm grasp on the obvious? Be careful. The mere fact that you walked into a health food store pretty much gets you better food, but it's not a guarantee.

Picture the novice perusing the food shelves of her local health food emporium: "I don't get it," she says. "It basically looks the same; the pasta is the same, just darker, the bread is the same, just heavier, the sauce is the same, just thicker."

It's basically true, but not entirely. The eggs are darker, usually, with harder shells and deeper-colored yolks. (You better test that at home.) The milk says "raw" (hopefully), and still has cream perched on top. The cereals are considerably more dense, so much so that they don't float away when the box is touched. The peanut butter has a thick layer of oil on top and requires considerable stirring to turn it into the real thing.

And there are new things, unlike anything on the supermarket shelves.

But as we follow her through the store, the biggest thing we notice is the size of her eyes, widening with every aisle. "I don't understand. Everything is more expensive!" And she's right.

You bet she's right, and thank heaven, because without those higher prices we wouldn't have these foods available at all. They cost more because they're different. The "heaviness," the "darkness," the "thickness," for the most part, means something important: these are real foods. (However, buyers need to beware everywhere.)

The idea is, foods have been sold to the masses for the profit and convenience of the food industry. Nearly all that you see on the shelves of a supermarket has been processed for shelf life, not your life. If it spoils, rots, bruises, goes stale, turns rancid, changes color, or tastes bad, it has to be thrown out, and that presents a little problem: You won't buy it. Not good for the bottom line. So they, uh, "do things," as we discussed in Section 1.

This is where the processing comes in. We know that foods are processed to accomplish a myriad of things: make more grow, make what grows grow larger, make it last longer, make it taste better, ship better, look better, cook better . . . yes, always better. Except better for you.

Someone has picked up on that, or there would be none of the more expensive health foods. Why pay more? Someone has picked up on the fact that all this processing for shelf life and cosmetics does nothing to make us healthier. The more the food is processed, the less it remains real food. The more it retains its vitality, the more you retain yours.

Having said that, we come to the most important part of buying this more expensive food: if you have decided to pay more, make sure you get what you pay for. Now our novice health nut shopper needs to remember the key rule of entering a health food store, which is, again: read the labels.

I wish I could say that a hundred more times, but nobody would stay and read it. In the more expensive foods, the profit margin would be that much higher if you could be made to pay more for a food that is not really worth more. The labels are vital here, since a few unscrupulous producers will try to take advantage of the knowledge that you already plan to pay a bit more in the first place.

Now that our novice has entered, and is reading, what does she look for? A little knowledge goes a long way, and it's not that tough.

- Flour is in many things. Make sure that it really is whole grain, if you've decided to pay more for it. In the case of wheat, it should say "100 percent stone ground whole wheat." Nearly everything else is cheating, such as "enriched," "100 percent unbleached enriched," even "100 percent stone ground wheat." You want the whole stuff, and with the least amount of preservatives possible. Bugs like the whole stuff, too, so get the freshest possible, refrigerate it, and use it up as quickly as possible.
- Avoid the words "partially hydrogenated." This is what makes the oils solid that make margarine, and they are often used in baked goods. Hydrogenation makes a chemical change in the oil that the body can't handle, so stay away from this if possible. Unfortunately, this is tough, as crackers, cookies, candy bars, and snack chips are hard to find without it. Sometimes you won't be able to avoid everything bad unless you graduate to really serious health nut status. In this day and age, even then it's tough.
- Raw milk and cheeses are good foods, within limits, assuming you can get them. There have been concerted efforts by the dairy industry to do away with raw products and have just the standard pasteurized, homogenized milk available. For an entertaining and informative little work on the subject, don't forget *The Milk Book,* by William C. Douglass, M.D.
- Even health foods have to taste reasonable, and the modern taste is sweet. So suppliers of health foods must compete, and they sometimes do it by sneaking in more sugar than you might think. Fructose may be a bit better than sucrose, but it's still sugar. Evaporated cane juice and dehydrated fruit juices are better because they at least have the original minerals from the sweetener, but they are still cheating tastewise. The weaker sweeteners, like rice syrup and malt syrup, are preferable. A neat

trick that pops up more than you might think is the use of multiple good sweeteners in the same item.

- Be very wary of sea salt, and its price. There are only two brands
I have found (see resource list) that leave the minerals in the
product, so nearly all "sea salts" are little better than common
table salt. (I have not found even one that is not mail order, but
things change daily. Look carefully!)

- Carob is far superior to chocolate as a food, if not in taste. It really isn't bad as a candy substitute because it requires less sugar
than chocolate by far. It's also low on the food allergy list. Most
of these confections still contain hydrogenated oils, but hey,
we're talking candy here.

- Fertile eggs, those that produce real chickens, are preferred.
How can you have healthy eggs from an unhappy hen?

- There is the same amount of oil in regular peanut butter as in
the health nut type. The difference is you can see the latter. It
does take some stirring to mix the good stuff, but it's worth it.
Homogenization is convenient, but it changes the chemical state
of the oil into an undesirable form. Store the good stuff in the
fridge, and use it up as quickly as possible, so the fats have less
time to go rancid. Try to remember that the popular brands are
also laced with sugar.

- Soups are nearly always better from the health food store. They
rarely have monosodium glutamate (MSG), which is worth
avoiding. Tin cans and other containers are superior to aluminum, which leaches into the food, but they are sometimes
hard to find.

- Try to get the date for when open-air bins of seeds, grains, trail
mix, etc., have been put out to avoid both the overgrowth of
mold and yeasts, and rancidity.

- Just because the produce is in a good store does not mean that
it's "organic." Such a word serves to drive the price way up.
Check with the manager if there is any question as to the source.
Real "organic" produce avoids insecticides, hormones, antibiotics, artificial fertilizers and other chemicals, and it's worth having—if you can really get it. There is also a certification process
involved, which helps. However, in packaged items one small

222 · **Nutritionally Incorrect**

part of the contents may be organic, while the rest is not. Watch the wording. Note that real organic foods do not look as good as the modern, genetically modified stuff.

- Do not buy something just because it says "low fat." This does not necessarily make it good. (In my opinion this is reason not to buy it, but this isn't the place for my anti-low-fat arguments.)

- Boxed and paper-sealed packages are better than aluminum or plastic, if available. The newer materials leach into foods. This affects both the taste and the body's toxin levels.

- Don't get overwhelmed. Consider picking a single area of interest at each visit, then concentrate on that, like cereals, produce, juices, or the like.

Drinks

This would be a nonsection for the full-blown health nut because the only true drink for the purist is water. That said, we can talk about the rest of the world:

- Water is, in fact, the only true drink; everything else is either liquid food, medicinal, or industrial waste, but that's another story. However, even health stores can carry less than ideal forms of water. Distilled water is for steam irons, not people, as it is lacking the all-important minerals that all natural waters possess. Look for deep-well sources of high mineral content water. Most labels are pretty clear on this type of thing.

- Plastic does leach into drinks from containers and should be avoided, especially with carbonated drinks, which are more reactive. Glass, if possible.

- Avoid aluminum containers for the same reason, except that the current findings on aluminum are scarier to me.

- Many health food store juices are loaded with added sugar, so know what you are getting, A frequent one is high-fructose corn sweetener, while the hardest to track down is concentrated fruit juice, the most common one being dehydrated grape. Since you're buying juice anyway, it's easy to miss this addition.

- The preferred juices are 100 percent juice, without the use of concentrates. Mixed is fine, just no concentrate.
- Vegetable juices are the best for you, though some take a little getting used to. The natural sugars in them metabolize more slowly than fruits, and they have more "phytogens," highly beneficial compounds.
- Try carrot juice. It's sweeter than most people think, and it's excellent for stomach problems.
- Some stores have local producers who supply fresh juices, not pasteurized. These are the best, but they must be drunk fairly quickly, before the taste turns.
- Some raw milk is supplied with the cream still on top. This is a plus, as most of it can be poured off and used separately.
- Raw milk does sour before pasteurized. Keep it chilled every moment for maximum shelf life.
- Rice milk, almond milk and oat milk are superior to regular (non-raw) milk, and they keep longer. Refrigerate them, even if the store does not. Soy milk may be okay for adults.
- Goat's milk is more like mother's milk than cow's milk. Both are naturally homogenized and lower in fat than cow's milk.
- Most herbal teas have no caffeine and many taste wonderful, even compared to regular tea. Instead of gambling, however, try a sampler pack, which only has three tea bags of each flavor.
- Herbal teas just for drinking require less sugar.
- Herbal teas for therapy can be very effective, but should be used with education, so read books specific to this area. Examples of good teas are ginger tea for nausea, and pau d'arco, or taheebo, for yeast; but there are many more.

Cosmetics

When people think of health food stores, usually cosmetics don't come to mind. Most good stores, however, have an impressive array, from toothpaste and deodorant to lines of hypoallergenic make-up.

There are good reasons to use them:

- Soaps that say "deodorant" or that they kill bacteria have no place on a person's skin. Chemicals that strong are bad for more than just the bacteria, and skin is absorptive. Though non-deodorant soaps are of course available elsewhere, well-chosen health store types include fat-soluble nutrients that are not only gentle, but also nourishing for skin. Read labels!
- Underarm deodorants are loaded with toxic chemicals. Adding antiperspirants is even worse because the anatomy in question is very absorptive. It's difficult to find a deodorant without aluminum in the "outside world"; it's harder to find one with it while cruising health food land. Even efforts to take advantage of the health craze by adding baking soda, etc., rarely includes removal of the bad stuff from popular brands.
- Toothpaste is the same story, different players. No matter what the party line is, fluoride is rat poison, plain and simple (no joke). If you take less of it, you only get less rat poison.

  This is a great time (now that you can adequately navigate) to float over to the book anchorage. Look for a book by John Yiamouyiannis called *Fluoride: the Aging Factor*. Adding peroxide and baking soda is great, but toothpaste without fluoride is just not available outside a health food store. Forget the sometimes emotional issue of fluoride; there's more. Besides tons of sugar, popular brands of toothpaste usually contain sodium lauryl sulfate. (I'm not sure what for.) This chemical has been implicated as an irritant in cases of canker sores (Wright 1998).

  Read labels (obviously a useful navigational tool) and get non-toxic toothpaste. Keep in mind that fluoride brands are available in store for those so inclined.
- No matter how they're priced, it's possible to find all sorts of cosmetic products having mineral oil as a major ingredient: hand lotions, facial creams, body oils, sun blocks, sun tan products, and I'll bet there are others. Mineral oil is cheap, very cheap. It also does a slick job (sorry) of getting absorbed into the skin very quickly. Very nice, except that it doesn't break down in there. It just sits around inhibiting the vitamin D process and helping your skin age. Avoid mineral oil whenever

possible. Checking out your local health food store is a good way to do it.

• Concerning makeup, (about which I know nothing) I spoke with a real, nonhealth food store, skin specialist. (They're now called "estheticians"!) She tells me that a few years ago it very much made a difference where you bought cosmetics, if health along with looking good made a difference. Now that the "health revolution" has occurred, there are many lines of cosmetics, nearly everywhere, that limit their products to truly natural, skin-pampering substances.

The only problem outside the health food store is knowing which lines are the healthy ones and which are just marketing hype, with a slick line about "natural," but cheaper materials. Most of the health store lines are made with some attention paid to natural concerns—not just a pretty face. For that reason you are probably better off at the health food store, unless you are very well informed about whatever outside brand you're using. I say again, read labels, and know what you're getting into—before it gets into you.

Devices

This is where you run into the neatest stuff. Some stores are loaded with more equipment than you see in Sears, while others have next to nothing. And the various types can be positively mind boggling. Health food stores have things you won't see anywhere else; there are some really unique devices, and devices can be anything. (Remember, a nuclear weapon isn't a bomb; it's a *device*.)

Some establishments may have tons of weight-lifting or bodybuilding gear and nothing else. Others, nothing for the he-man, but enough juicers and food processors to feed the five thousand with plenty to spare. This is where the real diversity of store owners shows in earnest.

Actually, one glance in a health food store and a whole philosophy leaps out at you. A store full of barbells is not the place to seek advice on wooden rollers for Chinese acupuncture points, and vice-versa. Just take one quick look . . . instant education.

Most stores, if they carry devices at all (I sure prefer the ones that do), can be divided into three very rough general classes: body-building, high-tech, and Eastern influence.

- **Body-Building:** I don't exercise this way, so this class has the least appeal for me, but the machines those guys use are worth ogling anyway. Unless you work out heavily, and at home, the bigger stuff may not appeal to you either. However, there can be some great little toys for the dreamer who actually thinks he'll stick with them on the couch, or who really believes that "only-three-minutes-a-day" will get him ready for the next Terminator audition. Still, great fun.

- **High-Tech:** These toys are commonly found in stores where more produce is carried. Food processors, juicers, peelers, dehydrators, water purifiers, yogurt makers, electric foot massagers, ozonators, digital scales, automatic blood pressure cuffs, head vibrators. I mean, you really can find some stuff.

  As you might imagine, the prices can be eye openers. A good food processor can set you back many hundreds of dollars, but often there will be a little manual job that slices, dices, peels, deals, rips, chips, chops, pops, shreds, and makes your bed, all for one low price.

  For the most part, these types of goodies will wait until the beginner is a bit more seasoned—less of a tourist. There is one exception, and that is water filters. There are water filters in every price range, and for every application. Only the absolutely most expensive, top-of-the-line models will take out fluoride (and you have to be careful even then), but all take out a large portion of particulate matter, and usually a fair amount of chlorine. Even the littlest camping filters are worth having. You never can tell, and you can't be too careful. Our municipal water is not to be trusted.

- **Eastern Influence:** If you find one of these types, drop anchor, you're in for a treat. This place displays all sorts of small, simple devices, usually of wood, beautifully hand-crafted, enticingly shaped, and thoroughly appealing to look at. And you'll have no idea what they're for. I love trying to figure them out. I guess that's part of the fun. In general, these widgets are in the realm of back-scratchers, muscle tension releasers, manual massage devices (there's that word again), tactile stimulation devices, acupuncture pressure point devices, qi enhancers, oriental puzzles and mind games, and often even more. They usually have to ask me to leave.

CHAPTER 22

Wait, Doc, Just a Few Questions . . .

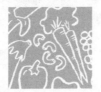

THE DOCTOR FINISHES his list of instructions: they've been written, they've been reviewed, they've been delivered. He rises to
leave the exam room. The patient seems content: no questions, no
concerns, no blank looks, no uncomfortable body language. Her
husband seems content as well. This session was so easy, so clear.
There is no hint of the occasional "eye roll" that a non-health-nut
spouse can give—the one that says, "That's Greek to me, and it
sounds no better in English."

This one will be different. No problem. The doorknob is within reach, and the doctor is now on the verge of beginning his first
on-time appointment in days. With knob in hand, it's only a few
more seconds to total success. "Hey, Doc, just a few questions."

It's amazing how many questions (good ones, too) come from
the person who appeared to have not the slightest interest in
what's going on. The world will always be blessed with those mad-
dening few who ask the same irrelevant question four times, but
usually the queries are legitimate and concerned.

I've long since learned that nutrition therapy sessions of instant
patient understanding are rare. It took me years to believe in real
nutrition and what it can do, but I thought I was just slower than

most. It also took way too long to recognize what to me was a significant axiom of health nut medicine: with health nut beginners the same twenty-five questions recur 90 percent of the time.

It's kind of like having a firm grasp on the obvious, as I look back. What's really frustrating is that after the years it took to appreciate the existence of the rule, it took years more to realize I should write the questions down! (Once I figured out the questions, at least I didn't wait years more to write down the answers.) It would have saved me tons of time.

Obviously, this rule implies that much of the information here is pretty basic, so you will find, unless you turned to this chapter first, that you already know many of the answers. In fact, you can use this chapter as a sort of starter info kit for those you might wish to educate, but who may not be willing to read a whole book. (Or believe any of it?)

Okay, so here they are, and you don't even need an office visit to get 'em.

1. What is nutrient density?

This is the general term that is implicit in several of the other questions. What you're looking for, as much as possible in the products you eat, are foods that have everything in them necessary for their own absorption and utilization by the body. If the carbohydrate, fat, or protein you just ate does not "self-contain" the items required by the body to handle that food, your body must take them from its own stored reserves.

These items can be enzymes, vitamins, minerals, fiber, or whatever else. Our body is expected to supply some things of its own, like acid, digestive enzymes, etc., but the idea is to keep the list as short as Mother Nature intended, to lessen biochemical stress. (See questions 2, 3, & 4.)

2. What is "refined" sugar, and what's the problem with eating it?

This is a major point, if not the major issue in the American diet, including all the furor about fat. Cane or beet juice, directly from the plant, is loaded with minerals and vitamins, all required for handling the sugar it supplies the body. The refining process removes or destroys all of these nutrients, leaving a white, crystalline chemical with an increased shelf-life—but no good for your life. You now have a nonfood substance that is much sweeter than anything for which the body was originally designed to handle.

Even honey (dark, raw honey) has enzymes, minerals and vitamins incorporated into its sugars. The pure white stuff, however, means you have a sweetener that is too strong for normal functioning of your pancreas, which must handle this sugar surge. This is accomplished by secreting insulin, an action that can be over-stimulated by refining. Plus, because refined sugar is devoid of nutrients itself, these must be supplied from other parts of your body to handle the refined chemical you just ate.

3. What is "refined" flour?

As you might imagine, this is similar to the refined sugar situation; that is, all the nutrients required for the utilization of the flour by the body are removed, leaving only pure, white starch. Flour is refined for shelf-life, again; this is wonderful because most bugs know better than to try to eat the stuff. Most humans, unfortunately, aren't so intelligent.

Besides removing nutrients, non-nutritive fiber is also removed. Though not absorbed, the fiber is important to the way the body handles the starch in the flour. Starch is considered a complex carbohydrate. Like sugar, it's in the carbohydrate class, but, unlike sugar, or simple carbohydrates, its sugars are linked together by chemical bonds into chains of sugar molecules. To get the sugar the body must break these bonds with digestive enzymes first. That is why starches do not taste sweet like simple sugars, since the process takes time.

Once the fiber is gone, however, the enzymes break down the starch to sugar faster than it could before the refining process occurred, which is another stress on the pancreas. This rapid release of sugar calories is part of our weight-gain problem in this country, since all this sugar must either be burned or stored (as fat, of course!). (An exception to this rule is adult diabetes, when the pancreas gets so stressed out that it screws up the handling of sugars and insulin, dumping sugar into the urine—not the ideal way to get rid of calories!)

By the way, don't be fooled by the advertising hype of the word "enriched." This is a trick and nothing more. Six synthetic vitamins (and low doses of those) are sprinkled in, and you are told your flour, bread, etc., is enriched. What a joke. Don't fall for this ploy, and don't forget you are also missing the fiber and all the minerals.

4. What are processed foods?

Anything that food companies have messed with is "processed." Unfortunately, unless you never eat fast food, do everything from your own garden, and eat it all fresh, you will end up with something frozen, sprayed, gassed, colored, flavored, preserved, pressed, emulsified, irradiated, sweetened, shipped unripe, or some such. Just do your best and let your nutritional supplements try to take up the slack for the nutritional sins you can't avoid committing.

This puts you right back into the nutrient density issue. (For review see questions 1, 2, and 3.)

5. What is wrong with chlorinated water?

Plenty. Chlorine is a highly reactive molecule (that's how it kills germs), and it continues its reactive ways inside us. I consider it highly toxic, to be respected and avoided, if possible. A frightening theory about the damage done by chlorine to the human body is laid out in the book *Coronaries/Cholesterol/Chlorine* by Joseph M. Price, M.D. It's beyond the scope of this book, but the basic premise is that chlorine reacts against the inner lining of our arteries to cause damage that the body must attempt to repair by its cholesterol-coating protection system that eventually gets out of hand by having too many scars to repair. (There's that cholesterol thing again.)

6. What can possibly be wrong with fruit juice?

Not all that much, but remember that fruit juice is concentrated fruit. You aren't eating edible skins or even the pulpy insides, so you are getting more concentrated sugars than you would get from the whole fruit. Also, fruit-juice companies sweeten many of their products with other juices so they will taste better and sell easier, and you can get a huge amount of calories here. Try to eat your fruit and drink your water. To lessen the high-level calorie load of simple sugars, dilute the juice with water as much as you can tolerate.

7. Are caffeine, nicotine, and alcohol really that bad?

Yes, at least the caffeine and nicotine are. Caffeine is an adrenal stimulant, which stresses the gland each time it is used. It won't kill you right away (in low doses, that is), but it is a definite long-term stressor. Nicotine is just plain toxic and addicting.

Alcohol, if used only in moderate doses, is probably not a problem, though recent research on pregnant women shows lower and lower doses seem to have problems attached.

8. Should I cut out red meat altogether?

Not necessarily, in my opinion. If you feel better off it, than cut it out. Some people seem to do better on small amounts, but I do not feel the human animal was meant to have large amounts. (We just couldn't run fast enough to catch much!) If you compare our intestinal tracts to those of pure carnivores and pure herbivores, you find that our systems seem to be somewhere in the middle.

Unfortunately, we have to deal with an additional situation today. The red meat we eat grazes on large amounts of vegetation that is in contact with all sorts of bug sprays and synthetic fertilizers, and these contaminants collect in the meat. Not only that, the animals themselves are given hormones to grow faster, in addition to the antibiotics they are given against diseases—more added toxic waste we don't need. Each additional chemical is another agent against which our body must defend, and for which it was not designed. Who's to say what the long-term effects are?

9. Can you avoid mixing proteins and carbohydrates?

Not completely. Many foods have protein, fat, and carbohydrates at the same time. However, the idea is to separate meats, cheeses, nuts, and seeds from the sweet things. The reason is that the stomach environment needs a more acid state (and more time) to break down protein and fat, while sugars require less acid and time to be digested. This is related to the rule (#15) to eat slowly and chew thoroughly, so that digestion can begin early. The idea is to help the body do its job as easily as possible, and decrease chemical stress as much as possible.

10. Why shouldn't I deep-fry foods?

Heat turns fats rancid very quickly, which is a toxic state, and even chemically changes the fat. (Not all fats are bad, no matter what they tell you on T.V.) Well-cooked fats can become generators of free-radicals, too, with which the body must deal. Soaking foods in liquid fat also increases its calorie content.

11. Are artificial sweeteners really that bad?

Yes. Your body thinks it's getting something sweet when it isn't. (It's not nice to fool Mother Nature.) Plus, there is increasing evidence that aspartame, the really popular sweetener called Nutra-Sweet™, is nowhere near as tame as we have been led to believe. It is reported to be the number-one source of complaints to the FDA to date, concerning adverse side effects.

There are other sweeteners, like FOS and stevia (an incredibly sweet herb that is not allowed to call itself a sweetener), that can be used as substitutes, but the artificial ones are a risk. The final work on Sucralose is not in yet, in my opinion, but I think this stuff deserves some respect.

12. How can you advise avoiding milk? What about calcium?

Let's deal with the second part first: you get your calcium in the same place the cows get it—green leafy plants.

Now, why actually avoid it? First of all, to demonstrate how I have a firm grasp of the obvious, let me say that cow's milk is for baby cows. They grow faster than we do, and they need more fat, among other things. Not only that, an adult cow will not drink milk; don't ask me why. (She must know something.)

Unfortunately, there's more: a calf will drink cow's milk, of course, but if it is pasteurized and homogenized, over time it will make the calf sick. Dairy farmers know better than to do it, they just don't always tell us about it. Homogenization is a big culprit here, as the process of busting up cream molecules to make them stay suspended in milk destroys at least one enzyme. This enzyme, xanthine oxidase, has been implicated as a cause of scarring in the human artery once it is chopped up. The significance of this is that the human body protects itself from such scarring by painting a thin layer of cholesterol on such damaged areas. (Interesting concept in this age of concern over cholesterol and blocked blood vessels.)

Milk, cream, butter, and cheese are not all bad. These products, purchased with the least amount of processing, can be very nutritious, as long as you are not allergic to them. An excellent book on the subject is *The Milk Book,* by William C. Douglass, M.D. Bear in mind, however, that certified raw milk is impossible to get in most places, thanks to the powers that be, telling us we need their help looking out for ourselves.

Also, be very careful with milk of any type in children under one year of age. Dairy allergies are not only extremely common, but they are also difficult to diagnose and easy to cause in the first year, in my opinion.

A secondary issue here is that of raw-milk cheese, and even goat cheese. These are only available in health food stores, unfortunately, but they are by far the best types in my opinion, though they tend to have a bit stronger taste.

13. Are there that many additives and are they all bad?

The number is positively mind boggling. Occasionally, vitamin C will be used as a preservative, or a truly natural color or flavor is added, but be very careful. Most additives are basically industrial chemicals that have no relationship to real foods whatsoever. Several nutritionists that I respect mention ingested food additives as being measured in pounds per year! (Ugh.)

14. Why do you say look for cravings; what's wrong with them?

Often nothing—just be aware that anything eaten every day, something "the day just doesn't seem complete without," may be an allergen, or sensitive food. You may be addicted to that food, such that eating it relieves symptoms for awhile. If you give up a food, and by day two to four you feel worse, continue the test for a week. You may end up feeling a whole lot better. Then you can test the food by eating it and looking for symptoms.

15. So, now what's the problem with aluminum cans?

It has long been known that aluminum in storage vessels leeches into foods contained within it, especially carbonated drinks (which rarely qualify as food!). What has more recently come to light is just how much aluminum actually ends up in the ingested material. It may be several thousand ppm (parts per million), far higher than is recognized as safe. It also doesn't take as long as previously thought for the process to occur. More evidence is being generated all the time over the link between aluminum, Alzheimer's Disease, and other problems associated with aging.

I always wondered why there has been a "freshness date" put on soft drinks, which have very little to keep fresh. At first I figured it was a ploy to sell more drinks. Now I wonder if there isn't another alternative, besides the concern as to whether we were getting the freshest carbonated water in town. The longer it sits on the shelf, the more aluminum it absorbs.

16. I always eat fast. What's the big deal?

Digestion starts in the mouth, with enzymes squirted from the salivary glands. (You didn't think it was just water!?) If this mixture is adequately combined, the rest of the job lower down has a huge head start. Plus, the time taken to chew food gives the body the stimulation to prepare more acid and enzymes to add to the digestive/absorptive process. Not only that, there are no teeth in the stomach, so the chewing you do up top is all you'll get. (Some animals actually swallow stones to help with the chewing process down lower in the digestive tract. I don't recommend it.)

17. What's wrong with grapes, dates, and figs?

Nothing, really, if you eat them sparingly. It's just that they carry a huge amount of sugar within them; natural, of course, but sugar just the same. That's a lot of calories. If you're going to have a candy bar, and you can substitute these fruits, do it, by all means, since they are loaded with minerals.

Remember, a raisin is a grape without the water, so you can really put away some calories in a hurry with a handful of raisins. Be careful. Even natural, unrefined calories are calories. Besides, dehydrating is a way of processing food. Though not always bad, you should respect and understand what the possible consequences are.

18. Must I eat organ meats?(!!)

No, only if you want to. (See question 24.)

19. Don't nuts and seeds have a lot of fat?

They have everything needed to grow a whole plant, so they are veritable powerhouses, including containing fats in differing amounts, plus a good quantity of protein. The raw fats (and we are talking about raw, fresh nuts and seeds) are excellent for killing your appetite—and for much longer than any sugar can. If you eat them slowly and chew thoroughly you can get some real, whole food in you without a lot of naked calories from sugar. Stay with fresh ones, as they can go rancid quickly.

20. How can you say that eggs are okay, after all their bad press?

That's because eggs are a wonderful food. Remember, everything needed to grow a living animal is contained within one. Most of the adverse publicity stems from the cholesterol issue, which is a long, sticky, somewhat political, and highly financial one. In my opinion, low-cholesterol diets are a bad idea in most cases. All of us need it, especially women, and if we do not eat it, our bodies will manufacture it. Many believe the manufactured form of cholesterol is more readily laid down in blood vessel walls. I tend to agree.

Besides, there is a limited amount of cholesterol you can absorb daily, no matter how much you eat, since there are a limited number of receptor sites in the body for that absorption.

Cholesterol, like all unsaturated fats, changes its form to a toxic one, when heated in the presence of air. Since the cholesterol is contained within the yolk of an egg, you should cook the egg without breaking the yolk sac. So, hard-boiled, soft-boiled, poached, "sunny-side," etc., are okay if the yolk stays intact. Scrambled or omelet-style, on the other hand, should be avoided.

If there are any questions concerning your personal cholesterol history, read more on the topic by authors like Carlton Fredericks, Linda Clark, Adelle Davis, Jonathan Wright, M.D., or Robert Atkins, M.D. (especially Dr. Atkins), and then talk with your health care practitioner about it.

Two final notes on the egg question: (1) Watch carefully when you introduce eggs to children; look for reactions; (2) Look for fertile eggs. (How can you expect the best eggs from an unhappy chicken?)

21. How do you find real whole-grain breads, pastas, cereals, etc.?

Some food co-ops have them, but basically you are left with the health food stores. The additional price is worth it. Some large grocery stores, however, are getting better. Beware of well-known brands trying to take advantage of unwary shoppers. They often use refined junk predominately, with a sprinkling of "whole-grain," which they promote heavily. Read labels carefully. A product must list its contents in descending order. Health Valley brand, though it often contains dried fruit, is becoming more prominent, and it is sweetened with fruit juice, while only using whole grains. Also, look for muesli-type cereals of lesser-known brands. Read labels!

22. Why is flaxseed oil beneficial?

Unprocessed (raw, cold-pressed) oils are the only way to go, as the heat (and other parts) of processing change the oils for the worse, nutritionally. Flaxseed and linseed oil are very high in essential fatty acids that other oils do not have, or have very little of. Flaxseed oil is involved in the work of Dr. Joanna Budwig, a German cancer researcher who has reported some amazing things with this lesser-known oil and its stabilizing effects on cell membranes.

23. What is carob, and why is it better than chocolate?

Carob is a cousin of chocolate. It is a bean, but, unlike cocoa, there is no caffeine. Also, the cocoa bean is extremely bitter, to the point of being inedible, requiring large amounts of sugar to sweeten it. Carob, while not actually sweet, is easily eaten raw, and requires minimal sweetening to make a desirable confection. It also causes far fewer sensitivity reactions. (No one can ever convince me that chocolate is not bad for skin!)

There is not much question that a milk chocolate bar is more desirable to a chocoholic, but carob may help in the withdrawal phase. The best candies are sweetened with dehydrated dates, instead of straight sugar. (See question 1) They also have a large assortment of types (plain, covered peanuts, almonds, raisins, rice cakes, etc.).

It's not a license to steal, but it is better for you than chocolate.

24. *What's the difference between calf and adult beef liver?*

If you're like me, you couldn't care less, but for those who like liver there is more to it than the fact that adult beef liver is tougher and tastes stronger. The liver is an important detoxifying organ, and the longer that an animal is alive, the longer its liver has to accumulate those toxins. Liver is a marvelous food, but if you are going to eat it, go for the young stuff. (Adelle Davis has some excellent information on the nutritional aspects of liver in her classic books, *Let's Eat Right To Keep Fit* and *Let's Get Well.*)

25. *Why give up foods for seven (or twenty-one) days?*

There is little doubt that food sensitivities are very real. To avoid controversy I avoid the word "allergy." It's possible to become sensitive to a food at any time (usually after eating it repetitively for extended periods), and it may even be a good food, so you are not limited to the junk food category. It's also common to be addicted to the food to which you are sensitive, due to the possibility that whenever the food is avoided the individual experiences withdrawal symptoms. Eating the item in question relieves the worst symptoms for awhile, but the problem persists.

It usually takes about seven days to clear the body of the effects of the sensitive food. Dairy may take up to twenty-one days. When you give it up, it must be given up completely. One crouton, while you are testing wheat, and you must start over for a legitimate test. Then, eat the food and evaluate whether you notice any symptoms (any, not necessarily the one you had originally). If symptoms occur, then again give up the item until clear and see if the food is really responsible. If not, then enjoy yourself!

If you give up a food and, during the first few days, you feel worse, then you are even more likely to be on the right track! You may want to tough it out and see if it clears. It may very well be withdrawal symptoms from something that has haunted you for years. If you confirm a suspect food, you may still be able to consume it from time to time (since it's probably a food you love). Avoid it for awhile, then see if it is tolerated once a week or so.

26. Is sugar really that big a deal?

Yes. (See questions 1 and 2)

Bibliography and Resource List

WE HAVE MENTIONED many sources of literature, supplements, and organizations throughout this book. They are all in this appendix, under their respective headings, plus others that are my concept of excellent choices for where to go next for additional information.

In many ways, you have barely scratched the surface with this book. Keep reading! This list is anything but exhaustive, but I know or have studied most of the names listed, and I recommend them as jumping-off points to greater understanding and better health.

Chapter 2

Sugar

www.holisticmed.com/aspartame/
www.holisticmed.com/splenda/
www.holisticmed.com/sweet/
The Aspartame Consumer Safety Network, http://web2.air-mail.net/marystod; 241-352-4268; P.O. Box 78064, Dallas, TX, 75738
Sugar Blues, William Dufty, Warner Books

Body, Mind & Sugar, E. M. Abrahamson, M.D. & A.W. Pezet, Avon Books

Sugar and Your Health, Ray C, Wunderlich Jr., M.D., Good Health Publishing

Low Blood Sugar and You, Carlton Fredricks, Ph.D., Grosset & Dunlap.

Honey (Note: These may be harder to find.)

Honey And Your Health, B.F. Beck, M.D., Bantam Books

Honey I Love You, Rev. Maurice Ness, Royal Publications

Chapter 4

Chlorine

Coronaries/Cholesterol/Chlorine. Joseph M. Price, M.D., Jove Publishing

Fluoride

"Lifesavers Guide to Fluoridation," Safe Water Foundation, 6439 Taggart Rd., Delaware, OH 43015

Fluoride: The Aging Factor, John Yiamouyiannis, Ph.D., Health Action Press

Pure Water Information

The Family News, 800-284-6263; 305-759-8710, www.family-healthnews.com

Ozone News of the International Ozone Association, 1331 Patuxent Dr., Ashton, MD 20861; "203-348-3542; 203-967-4845 (F); www.int-ozone-assoc.org

Water Filters

Multipure Corp., 800-622-9206, 702-360-8880, www.multi-pure.com

Everpure Corp., 800-942-1153, 630-654-4000, www.everpure.com

Chapter 5

MSG

In Bad Taste: The MSG Syndrome, George R. Schwartz, M.D., Signet Books

Milk Processing
The Milk Book, W.C. Douglass, M.D., Second Opinion
    Publishing

Chapter 6

Antibiotic Overuse
The Yeast Connection Handbook, William G. Crook, M.D.,
    Professional Books
Hormone Overuse
The Yeast Connection and the Woman, William G. Crook,
    Professional Books
Yeast
The Yeast Connection Handbook, William G. Crook,
    Professional Books

Chapters 7–8

The Need for Vitamins
The Real Vitamin & Mineral Book, Shari Lieberman, Ph.D.,
    R.D., & Nancy Bruning, Avery Publishing
Vitamin B6
Vitamin B6: The Doctor's Report, John Ellis, M.D. & James
    Presley, Harper & Row
Vitamin E
Your Child and Vitamin E, Wilfred E. Shute, M.D., Keats
    Publishing

Chapter 9

Vitamin C
The Healing Factor, Irwin Stone, Grosset & Dunlap
*Cancer and Vitamin C: A Discussion of the Nature, Causes,
    Prevention, and Treatment of Cancer with Special Reference
    to the Value of Vitamin C,* Evan Cameron, F.R.C.S., & Linus
    Pauling, Ph.D., Camino Press
Every Second Child, Archibald Kalakerinos, M.D., Keats
    Publishing

Other excellent authors on vitamins and other nutrition topics, with names well worth remembering, are Frederick Klenner, M.D., Robert Cathcart, M.D., William C. Douglas, M.D., and Robert Atkins, M.D.

Chapter 10

Amino acids

Carlson Wade's Amino Acids Book, Carlson Wade, Keats Publishing

The Healing Nutrients Within, Eric R. Braverman, M.D., with Carl C. Pfeiffer, M.D., Ph.D., Keats Publishing

Herbs

Herbally Yours, Penny C. Royal, Sound Nutrition Publishing

Earl Mindell's Herb Bible, Earl Mindell, Ph.D., R.Ph., Simon & Schuster

The Herb Book, John Lust, Bantam Books

Chapter 12

Homeopathy

Everybody's Guide To Homeopathic Medicines, Cummings and Ullman, J.P. Tarcher/Putnam

Discovering Homeopathy, Dana Ullman, J.P. Tarcher/Putnam

The Consumer's Guide to Homeopathy, Dana Ullman, M.Ph., J.P. Tarcher/Putnam

Homeopathic Medicine at Home, Jane Heimlich, Maesimund B. Panos, Robert Mendelsohn, J.P. Tarcher/Putnam

Chapter 13

Fatigue

Solved: The Riddle of Illness, Stephen E. Langer, M.D., James F. Scheer, Keats Publishing

Chronic Fatigue Syndrome and the Yeast Connection, William G. Crook, M.D., Professional Books, Jackson, TN

The Yeast Connection, William G. Crook, Vintage Books

Chapter 14

Weight control

The New Atkins Diet Revolution, Robert Atkins, M.D., Bantam
Solved: The Riddle of Illness, Langer & Scheer, Keats Publishing
Dr. Atkins' Diet Revolution, Robert C. Atkins, M.D., Bantam
Hypothyroidism: The Unsuspected Illness, Broda Barnes, Ty
    Crowell Company
Sugar Busters, Morrison C. Bethea, Samuel S. Andrews,
    Steward H. Leighton, Ballantine Books

Chapter 15

Coenzyme Q10

The Miracle Nutrient: Coenzyme Q10, Emile G. Bliznakov,
    M.D., & G. L. Hunt, Bantam Books

Chapter 16

Constipation

Hypothyroidism: The Unsuspected Illness, Broda Barnes, Ty
    Crowell Company
Solved: The Riddle of Illness, Langer & Scheer, Keats Publishing

Chapter 17

Progesterone

Natural Hormone Replacement, J. Wright, MD, & J.
    Morgenthaler, Smart Publications, P.O. Box 4667, Petaluma,
    CA, 800-543-3873; fax: 707-769-8016;
    www.smart-publications.com

Lotions

    Mill Creek (in health food stores)
    Nature's Gate (in health food stores)
    Rejuvenex (www.lef.org, 800-544-4440, 954-766-8433)

Chapter 18

Behavior

Is This Your Child? Doris Rapp, M.D., Wm. Morrow & Company, Inc.

Allergies and the Hyperactive Child, Rapp, M.D., Simon & Schuster.

The Feingold Cookbook for Hyperactive Children, Ben F. Feingold, M.D., & Helene S. Feingold, Random House

Feed Your Kids Right, Lendon Smith, M.D., Dell Books

Help for the Hyperactive Child, William G. Crook, M.D., Professional Books

Solving the Puzzle of Your Hard-To-Raise Child, William G. Crook, M.D.

Common Questions on Schizophrenia and Their Answers, Abram Hoffer, M.D., Ph.D., Keats Publishing

How To Live with Schizophrenia, Abram Hoffer, Osmond, & Kahan, Revised by Citadel Press, NY

Mental and Elemental Nutrients, C. Pfeiffer, MD, Keats Publishing, New Canaan, CT

Great Smokies Diagnostic Laboratories, Asheville, North Carolina, 800-522-4762, 828-253-0621, www.gsdl.com"

Omegatech Laboratory, Troutdale, Virginia, 800-437-1404, 440-835-2150, www.kingjamesomegatech-lab.com

Doctor's Data, Chicago, Illinois, 800-323-2784, 630-377-8139, www.doctorsdata.com

Chapter 19

Older and Wiser

Dr. Atkins' Health Revolution, Robert C. Atkins, M.D., Bantam Books

Senility

Smart Nutrients: A Guide to Nutrients That Can Prevent and Reverse Senility, Abram Hoffer, M.D., M. Walker, D.P.M., Avery Publishing Group

Arthritis

The Arthritis Cure, Jason Theodosakis, M.D., Saint Martin's Press

There Is a Cure For Arthritis, Paavo Airola, N.D., Parker
  Publishing

Chapter 20
Salt
The Grain & Salt Society, Inc.
273 Fairway Drive
Asheville, North Carolina 28805
800-TOP-SALT (867-7258), 828-299-9005
www.celtic-seasalt.com

Redmond Minerals, Inc.
P.O. Box 219
Redmond, Utah 84652
800-367-7258, 435-529-7402
www.realsalt.com

Therapeutic Nutrition

I believe the best general reference on nutritional therapies has
to be *Prescription For Nutritional Healing* by James Balch, M.D.,
& Phyllis Balch, C.N.C., Avery Publishing Group. It has been
recently revised, and contains recommendations, in order of
importance, for hundreds of symptoms and diseases. This is a
must!

Dr. Wright's Guide to Healing With Nutrition, Jonathan V.
  Wright, M.D., Rodale Press.
Nutrition, Health & Disease, Gary P. Todd, M.D., Donning
  Publishers, Norfolk, Virginia.
Putting It All Together: The New Orthomolecular Nutrition, A.
  Hoffer, M.D., Mort Walker, D.P.M., Keats Publishing.
Alternative Medicine: the Definitive Guide, compiled by the
  Goldberg Group, Future Medicine Pub, Puyallup, WA.

Newsletters

My selection for the finest nutrition newsletter around is called *Nutrition and Healing* by Jonathan V. Wright, M.D. It is worth every penny, every month. Call 800-851-7100 or 978-287-2237. (Remember the names Wright and Alan Gaby. These guys are the gold standard for therapeutic nutrition.)

Also consider *Health and Healing* by Julian Whittaker, M.D. This started as a great mouthpiece for correcting heart disease problems without surgery, but has since become a magnificent general nutrition therapy source. Call 800-777-5005; 301-340-2100; www.drwhitaker.com.

Another excellent newsletter is *Second Opinion* by Robert Rowen, M.D. Call 800-728-2288; 770-399-5617.

Last, and hopefully not least, is my own newsletter: To Your Health. Call 800-851-7100 or 978-287-2237.

General Nutrition

The Real Vitamin & Mineral Book, Shari Lieberman, R.D., Ph.D., Nancy Bruning, Avery Publishers. This is the low-down on great nutrition from the king (oops, queen) of dietitians.

Hoffer's Law's of Natural Nutrition, Abram Hoffer, M.D., Ph.D., Quarry Press, Kingston, ON.

There are *many* others, and I mean really good ones. I recommend you read everything you can get your hands on, then you decide what is reasonable. Classic authors are Adelle Davis, Linda Clark, Carlton Fredricks, and Richard Passwater.

On the Internet

The Weston A. Price Foundation: www.westonaprice.org; westonaprice@msn.com; 202-333-HEAL; fax: 202-333-0002

The Price-Pottenger Nutrition Foundation: www.price-pottenger.org; 800-FOODS-4-U; 619-462-7600; fax: 619-433-3136

The Life Extension Foundation: www.lef.org; 800-841-5433; 954-766-8433; fax: 954-761-9199

The Health Sciences Institute: www.healthsciencesonline.com; 819 N. Charles Street, Baltimore, MD 21201; 978-514-7852 (U.S.); 978-514-7857; 410-230-1273 (F).

The Holistic Healing Web Page: www.holisticmed.com

Cookbooks

I'm not sure there is a perfect place to go for recipes. Unfortunately, I'm not the best person to ask in terms of taste because I usually burn the salad. However, here are my ideas for some of the best ways to go:

Nourishing Traditions: The Cookbook That Challenges Politically Correct Nutrition and the Diet Dictocrats, Sally Fallon, Pro Perkins Publishing. If you aren't hung up on the current hype about cholesterol and animal fat, this is the way to go. (I love the title . . . wish I'd thought of it.)

The Good Breakfast Book, Nikki & David Goldbeck, Ceres Press.

Whole Foods for the Whole Family, Roberta B. Johnson (ed.), NAL/Dutton (a La Leche League Publication) 708-519-7730, fax 708-519-0035. This is well-indexed, and good for the "it's 4 o'clock, what to make?!" syndrome. It's also not overwhelming for the beginner health nut in the kitchen.

The Yeast Connection Cookbook, William G. Crook, M.D., Marjorie Hurt Jones, R.N., Professional Books, Jackson, TN. If yeast ends up being a problem in your history, this baby is invaluable. For just plain healthy recipes, it's still great.

The Feingold Cookbook for Hyperactive Children, Ben F. Feingold, M.D., and Helene S. Feingold, Random House. If you or your family members have any chemical sensitivities, this is a must. It is also a compendium of healthful recipes for everyone.

Let's Cook It Right, Adelle Davis, Harcourt, Brace & World. This is the original classic, but still around, and worth the search.

Also recommended is a trip to the public library or the Internet. Look up "cookbooks." Select recipes you might like, test them, copy them, keeping only the ones you like. This way is probably the most economical, obviously, especially when the recipes are different enough that you really might not make them more than once!

Physicians

Possible sources of local physicians open to these approaches are potentially available from:

1. The National Health Federation (NHF), at 818-357-2181, FAX 818-303-0642;

2. The American College of Advancement in Medicine (ACAM), at 800-532-3688; 949-583-7666; www.acam.org

3. The International Bio-Oxidative Medicine Foundation (IBOM), P.O. Box 13205, Oklahoma City, OK 73113;

4. The American Academy of Environmental Medicine (AAEM), at 316-684-5500; fax: 316-684-5709; www.aaem.com; administrator@aaem.com

5. A great source of information for all sorts of health questions, including local sources of physicians: Life Extension Foundation, at 1-800-841-5433; 954-766-8433; fax: 954-761-9199; www.lef.org.

Index

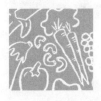

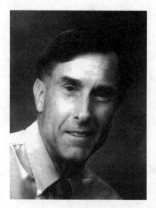

About the Author

A nutritionally oriented medical doctor
in practice for over a decade, Dr. Spreen
is known for his Nutrition Physician™
website, which offers nutrient therapy
information directly to the public.
Author of *Smart Medicine* and *The
Menopause Diet,* he wears a second hat
as a coach of competitive divers at the
national and Olympic levels.

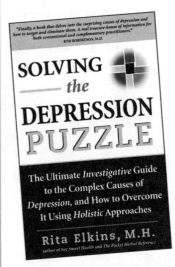
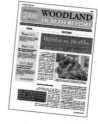